"Regardless of having worked in the area of fluency for 5 years, I continue to be surprised by the insensitivity and injustices to which people who stutter are subjected. I have known Lise since 1991, and have followed the progression of her son's stuttering and therapy. I always sympathized with her, as I do with all families in such situations, but I did not realize until reading this book the number of challenges faced by Lucas and his family. Unfortunately, they are not alone. It is my hope that society will come to recognize stuttering for what it is, but also what it is not. Lise has shown much courage in exposing her and her son's private moments, sharing the joy and frequent hardship which accompany this disorder. She also takes the reader one important step further by providing practical suggestions and advice to parents and teachers."

– Karen Luker, B.A., M.H.Sc.
Speech-Language Pathologist

"Living and Learning With a Child who Stutters affords the reader a sensitive and personalized glimpse into the daily problems and frustrations encountered by a child who stutters and the efforts of a caring family to help him cope. Parents will identify. Professionals will be reminded of long-standing gaps in service for children who stutter and of the need to advocate for improvements within their respective work milieus. All readers will appreciate this book for the insight and learning experience it provides."

– Terrence J. Laughlin, Ph.D., C.Psych., Psychologist
Chief of Psychological Services for the Ottawa Board of Education

"Having grown up as a child who stuttered severely, and as an adult who, while I have been fairly successful in coping with my problem, nevertheless still have to contend with it, I can comment from my own experience on Mrs. Cloutier-Steele's account. I have been aware of the author's work since seeing a very informative and sensitive TVOntario program on stuttering, which prompted me to write to her and compliment her on her efforts to gain better understanding for those of us who stutter, but particularly for children who are subjected to all sorts of painful stresses due to ignorance and insensitivity. This personal account of sufferings, and also the achievements of a child who stutters and of his family certainly rings true. I have no hesitation in recommending it as valuable reading both for the parents of children who stutter, and for professionals such as teachers who need to develop a sensitive understanding of stuttering."

– David Radcliffe, Ph.D., Associate Dean, Faculty of Education
University of Western Ontario

"I have just finished reading Living and Learning With a Child who Stutters *and found it a sensitive, honest portrayal of the trials and heartaches facing parents of stuttering children. At times humorous, at times tragic, the book documents a mother's quest to ensure that her stuttering son receive both a quality education and the best speech therapy possible. As strange as it may seem, in these modern times, the most basic right of a good education and quality special services all too often are not readily attainable for parents of children who stutter. Teachers administrators and, unfortunately, many speech-language pathologists are unaware of the impact stuttering has on a child's educational and social progress. My hope is that Mrs. Cloutier-Steele's experience will encourage the rest of us to increase our efforts on behalf of children who stutter and their parents."*

– Carl W. Dell Jr., Ph.D., Speech-Language Pathologist
Associate Professor, Eastern Illinois University

LIVING AND LEARNING WITH A CHILD WHO STUTTERS

"From a Parent's Point of View"

LISE G. CLOUTIER-STEELE

NC PRESS LIMITED
TORONTO, 1995

Photograph of Lise G. Cloutier-Steele by The Bay, Ottawa.
Front cover photograph by David Lancaster.
Back cover photograph of the film crew and the author's family,
left to right: Jonathan, Lise, Lucas with their dog Cooper, David,
Paul, Jim, Peter and Vladimir.
Cover Design by Gerry Ginsberg.

Canadian Cataloguing in Publication Data

Main Entry under title:
Cloutier-Steele, Lise G. (Lise Ginette), 1952-
    Living and learning with a child who stutters

(FAMILYbooks)
ISBN 1-55021-094-7

1. Stuttering in children. 2. Speech therapy for children. I. Title.
RJ496.S8C56 1995   618.92'8554   C95-931200-5

We would like to thank the Ontario Arts Council, the Ontario
Publishing Centre, the Ontario Ministry of Culture, Tourism
and Recreation, the Ontario Development Corporation, the
Canada Council and the Government of Canada, Department
of Canadian Heritage and the Association for the Export of
Canadian Books, for their assistance in the production and mar-
keting of this book.

New Canada Publications, a division of NC Press Limited,
Box 452, Station A, Toronto, Ontario, Canada, M5W 1H8.

Printed and bound in Canada

CONTENTS

Dedication

To the memory of our friend Marie Poulos

"The whole area of stuttering has suffered from the apathy and ignorance of the medical and teaching professions and their lack of understanding of the difficulties raised by dysfluency in group situations, the acute pain of social censure from childhood onwards, and the destruction of lives by society's attitudes. The time has come for changes in the attitude of politicians, educators, doctors and the general public towards people who stutter. It is long overdue . . . "

– Jock Carlisle, Ph.D
Scientist and Author of TANGLED TONGUE

ACKNOWLEDGEMENTS

My sincere thanks go out to the following individuals and treatment centre for their significant contributions to *Living and Learning with a Child Who Stutters*: **Sally Bowman**, Associate Professor Emeritus of Speech Pathology, author of *Everything You Should Know About Stuttering*, Indiana University's School of Medicine (U.S.A.), **Jock Carlisle**, Ph.D., author of *Tangled Tongue*, **David Radcliffe**, Associate Dean, Faculty of Education, The University of Western Ontario, **Margo** of Sarnia, Ontario, **Bob Ireland**, Assistant Superintendent, the Metropolitan Separate School Board, Toronto, Ontario, **Paula Moss**, B. Med. Sci, Hons, Speech-Language Pathologist, Willowdale, Ontario, **William G. Webster**, Ph.D., co-author of *Facilitating Fluency*, Brock University, St. Catharines, Ontario, **Douglas H. Fullerton**, O.C., M. Com., LL.D., D.U.C., Ottawa, Ontario, The **Communications Disorders Department** of the Rehabilitation Centre, Ottawa, Ontario, **Carl Dell Jr.**, Ph.D., Speech-Language Pathologist, author of *Treating the School-aged Stutterer*, Speech and Hearing Clinic, Eastern Illinois University (U.S.A.), **Janice Westbrook**, Ph.D., M.Ed., CCC-SP, Editor of *The Staff*, Garland, Texas (U.S.A.) and **David Forster**, M.Sc., for his invaluable scientific input.

I am equally grateful to the five specialists who reviewed my manuscript: **Terrence J. Laughlin**, Ph.D., C.Psych., Chief of Psychological Services, the Ottawa Board of Education, **Selwyn M. Smith**, M.D., F.R.C.P.C., F.A.P.A., Ottawa, Ontario, **Karen Luker**, M.H.Sc., SLP(C), Ottawa, Ontario, **David Radcliffe**, Associate Dean, Faculty of Education, The University of Western Ontario, and to **Carl Dell Jr.**, Ph.D., Speech-Language Pathologist, Speech and Hearing Clinic, Eastern Illinois University (U.S.A.). Thanks to their friendship and support, I completed a special project of which I am very proud.

To my parents, my brother and to my friends Gay Kerr, John Ahlbach, Executive Director of the National Stuttering Project, San Francisco, California, Gaye Thompson, Gary Vienneau, George Shields, the Ontario Barber Shop Singers, Mireille Landry, Paul Richer and Joyce Sharp, I wish to say thank you for your help and your words of encouragement over the years.

Special thanks to my eldest son Jonathan for his free spirit and his ability to make me laugh (even when I don't feel like it), and to my husband Paul for sharing his life with me and my boys.

Finally, my most sincere thanks to Lucas for agreeing to let me tell his story in the hope that it will be helpful to other children like him and their parents.

PROLOGUE

Living with a child who stutters continues to be a learning experience for me. Over the years, I have found ways to cope with my son Lucas' disability, but there have been times when it was difficult. I knew from the start that I would have to inform myself in order to be of any help to my child. I remember feeling so helpless when he first started to stutter; this problem was much bigger than a scraped knee! I couldn't understand why he suddenly started to stutter and, as many other mothers like me have admitted, I too, felt partly responsible for my son's dysfluent speech.

From age 3 to 4, the impediment in Lucas' speech was not always present. He would stutter for a few weeks at a time, and then be fluent for the next month. The intermittent speech dysfluency made it next to impossible for his pediatrician to identify the disorder as my son seemed to be having a good speech day whenever a medical appointment had been scheduled. Back home we went. And yes, I was tempted to ask Lucas why he didn't stutter when he was supposed to!

Although most of the children who begin stuttering at a young age outgrow the condition in a few months, particularly the girls, my son was to develop a confirmed stuttering pattern. If you have a child who stutters, or if you are the teacher of a dysfluent student, it is important to know that specialists now believe that early intervention with speech therapy can help prevent stuttering from becoming a life-long affliction. Don't wait for the stuttering to go away on its own, or until the child develops erratic speech patterns which may be harder to undo. Take the necessary steps to have an assessment done by a qualified speech-language pathologist as soon as possible.

My son will soon be 16 years old. At age ten, he was a graduate of the *Precision Fluency Shaping Program (PFSP)*, a intensive treatment opportunity offered to adults and adolescents at the Rehabilitation Centre of the Royal Ottawa Health Care Group, Ottawa (CANADA). He had done well with the program, and he was proud of his newly-acquired speech skills. He was free at last to speak his mind and his sentences seemed to flow so easily. Maintaining his techniques, however, was not an easy thing for him to do.

Parents and teachers should know that regardless of age, when a patient acquires the speech skills to control the stutter, he or she must work at it each and every day, otherwise, there will be a relapse. Lucas has had several breakdowns in his speech during the past four years, but he was always able to get himself back on track with maintenance therapy. Unfortunately, now that he has entered adolescence, he has gone into complete denial, a situation I will discuss later in this book.

I'm told this is very typical of teenagers who stutter, however, I can't help but wonder how many more phases of stuttering will we have to go through. I say we because not only has Lucas' stutter had a dramatic impact on his daily activities, but in many ways, some good and some bad, it has also altered our life as a family.

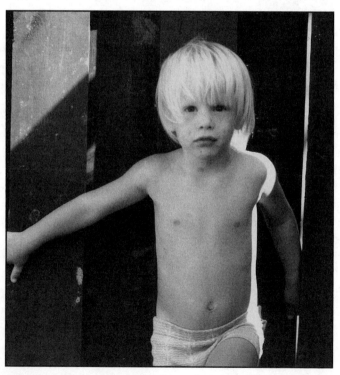

Lucas started to stutter at age 3.

CHAPTER 1

WHAT IS STUTTERING?

Before I introduce the first story I wrote about my son Lucas, I would like to discuss what stuttering is all about. By doing so, I hope to clear up whatever misconceptions the reader may have about people who stutter.

Over the years, I had the opportunity to observe the reactions of people with whom my son came into contact. Many were considerate and kind while others seemed to be either afraid of, or uncomfortable with, his stutter. It wasn't until recently that I came to the conclusion that those who experienced discomfort at the sound of the bumps in his speech were almost always inclined to believe he wasn't as bright as the other children. What many didn't know was that people who stutter are just like you and me, except of course, for the physical difficulties they experience when they speak.

There were times when I found myself talking (most likely complaining) to my son's personal speech-language pathologist about the lack of written material on stuttering in our Canadian book stores, libraries and school systems. One day, she gave me a copy of a small booklet she had obtained through Bowman Associates of Indianapolis, Indiana. This publication was appropriately titled *What Everyone Should Know About Stuttering* and was written by Sally Bowman, Associate Professor Emeritus of Speech Pathology, Department of Otolaryngology, Head and Neck Surgery at Indiana University's School of Medicine.

Although Professor Bowman wrote her booklet several years ago, her words paint an accurate picture of what the general public still thinks about people who stutter, and on how dysfluent people view themselves. I am grateful to Professor Bowman for granting me permission to reproduce her material in Chapter 1 of my book in the hope that many will find the information very useful. But first, let me tell you a bit more about this fluency specialist and author.

She has served as Advisor to the Indiana Council on Stuttering since 1972. The author of numerous video tapes and publications, Professor Bowman has made many contributions to the field of speech-language pathology. Among her many accomplishments is the founding and directing of an annual speech camp for children who stutter held in Indianapolis, Indiana. *(For more information about Sally Bowman's speech camp, see Reference Guide.)*

What is stuttering?

It is a disorder in which the flow of continuous speech is interrupted by repetition or prolongation of a word, a syllable, or a sound. It is a disorder of timing, of not being able to perform the motor sequence of a sound at the proper moment. It is often accompanied by the learned accessory behaviours of avoidance and struggle. It is sometimes accompanied by silent gaps and tremor. It is a set of learned behaviour patterns or an organic or neuromuscular disorder, NOT neurosis.

What does the general public think about people who stutter?

Through the years, people have developed some incorrect stereotypes about people who stutter . . . that they are nervous, funny, have a bad habit, are crazy, not bright, or that their teacher made them switch from left-handed to right-handed.

What have been some of the treatments tried for stuttering?

Throughout history, people who stutter have been subjected to many types of therapy such as bathing, ventriloquism training, electric shock, Swedish massage, exercise, hypnosis, psychotherapy, acupuncture, surgery, technical devices.

[As reported by Sally Bowman, there were 60 machines for curing stuttering registered with the U.S. Patent Office at the time of publication of her booklet. Other inventions have undoubtedly been added to the list in recent years, and I know of a couple registered with the Canadian Patent Office.]

People who stutter have also had to endure punishment, knitting needles forced through their tongues, chewing garlic, institutionalization, having grass fibres burned on their skin, leeches on their lips, their tongues slit or burned, drinking such concoctions as persimmon stones, raw eggs, charred frog tongues and goat feces.

How are people who stutter treated by others around them?

Autobiographies written by people who stutter show that they have been teased by their sisters and brothers, slapped and punished by their parents, mocked and laughed at by friends and strangers, blamed for family conflicts, forced to eat in the kitchen when company came, made to feel lonely and isolated or over-protected and spoiled.

How do people who stutter view themselves?

Dysfluent people feel quite normal except when they are speaking, but the attitudes and evaluations of those around them help form their self-concepts. If a person who stutters is made to feel different, s/he may spend extra time on extreme and careful grooming, join only groups that are more tolerant, choose a career where speech is not important (an accountant or a computer programmer, for example), or where s/he doesn't stutter (a singer or an actor), stick to small talk only or assume an accent or dialect or be loud and laugh a lot or be habitually silent.

What are the main characteristics of stuttering?

As with hearing loss, asthma, allergies and many other conditions, early and mild stuttering may be difficult to diagnose. Two of the chief characteristics are *Repetition* and *Prolongation*. Two other prominent characteristics of stuttering are the *Silent Gap*, also known as *Blockage* and *Tremor*.

How do people who stutter react to moments of stuttering?

Emotionally, with fear of pity, social penalty, listener loss, humiliation, embarrassment, rejection, shame, guilt, hostility, frustration, inability to communicate and silence. Physically, with shifts to the falsetto voice, extreme exhalation, shifting of the lips and jaw to the side, increase in blood pressure, pulse rate, muscle tension and dilation of pupils.

What causes some people who stutter to feel fearful?

Usually, the situation fears come first . . . listeners who are impatient, irritated, pitying, hostile or rejecting the content and implication of the message, specific settings, such as a store, airport, doctor's office, telephone calls, confrontations with authority, such as a teacher, parent or employer, reading aloud, giving his/her name and address.

Then, the fear of the sound, syllable or word occurs as the person who stutters gathers his/her thoughts . . . the position of the word in the message, certain words, phrases or syllables, more fear of nouns, adjectives and verbs because they have more meaning . . . generally more fear on words with initial consonants, more fear on initial sounds of accented syllables or long words, and more fear of sounds in the dominant syllable.

How do people who stutter cope when they anticipate stuttering?

People who are dysfluent will try almost anything to prevent stuttering. Many maintain a constant vigilance and revision of strategies. One of the most frequent techniques is the use of *Postponement* and *Avoidance* methods . . . uses "ah," "eh," "um," "yeah," *[my son Lucas currently uses "yo"]* "you know," "well" . . . silently rehearses feared words, swallows, licks lips, coughs, yawns, laughs, grinds teeth, starts to speak, then pretends to stop and think, lets the listener finish the sentence, substitutes or adds words to the original thought, refuses to enter a conversation or to attempt certain words. Some people who stutter develop very large vocabularies because of their need for substitution words.

Do these avoidance techniques work?

No. The constant vigilance to prevent stuttering becomes so unbearable that stuttering occurs sooner or later. And, once these techniques become automatic, some people who stutter will begin to have trouble with starter words or substitution words they have devised.

How do people who stutter cope after stuttering begins?

By developing one or more learned *struggle behaviours*, such as gasping, sniffing, grunting, snorting, gagging, speaking on inhaled air, panting, teeth grinding, eye blinking, facial grimaces, tongue protrusion, jerking the body, head or jaw, finger snapping, lip smacking, feet stomping, hand slapping, fist clenching, whistling or feet tapping.

What makes dysfluent people adopt such strange struggle behaviours?

This variety of learned behaviours differs from one person to another, but basically, some of these gestures help to open or close the airway or voice box. Sometimes they occur automatically as frustration and fear of rejection increases and some seem to be learned by chance and coincide with tremor. Eventually, these behaviours become automatic. *Do these struggle behaviours help?* No. These reactions also interrupt the continuous flow of speech and increase the discomfort of the listener and the person who stutters.

Do all dysfluent people react to situations the same way?

Just as there is no single sound or class of sounds more difficult for all people who stutter, so are their reactions to given widely varied situations. This variability is probably due to the different learning experiences in their backgrounds. Patterns may differ with different people who stutter; some have difficulty with memorized material and reading, some speak better when their listener is hostile or impatient, some speak better when speaking slowly, some are better when they speed up their speech, some have more difficulty when they are ill, some speak better when they are tired, some have normal EEG's, some have a family history of the disorder, some have more difficulty when they are tense, and some speak better under the influence of alcohol or medication.

What is the incidence of stuttering?

It is universal, and affects 4% of the general population, declining to 1% after preschool years. It affects three times as many males as females, and it usually begins before 5 years of age. Stuttering is higher among younger age groups. In childhood, it usually consists of whole word repetitions and prolongations without struggle behaviour. Rarely does sudden onset of stuttering occur in adults as a result of head trauma or stroke.

Does stuttering occur on every word?

No. It is intermittent. And, there is marked reduction or even absence of stuttering when the person sings, whispers, speaks in rhythm, shadows, speaks in chorus or speaks in delayed auditory feedback (fluency aid).

How is stuttering treated today?

Stuttering is a highly complex, unsolved scientific problem and is now considered a clinical disorder. The profession of speech pathology has made great strides in updating old ideas and practices regarding the diagnosis and treatment of stuttering.

*   *   *

Due to the many time pressures we face on a daily basis, the majority of us tend to speak at a rate which is much too fast. There are also times when we don't pay enough attention to what is said. If you do meet a person who stutters, please remember to be patient. An attentive listener can help a dysfluent person communicate with less difficulty and struggle.

Except for one specific instance where I am quoting from a document made public many years ago, the reader will notice that the word *stutterer* has been avoided throughout the book. The fact that someone stutters does **NOT** define what they are.

CHAPTER 2

THE EARLY SCHOOL YEARS

The first story I wrote about my son was essentially one of frustration. From pre-kindergarten to Grade 5, Lucas attended two different schools under the jurisdiction of one school board in Ottawa, Ontario, and the experience proved to be as difficult for me as it was for him. In recent years, I have spoken to dozens of other parents living across our province, who related similar experiences.

The following is not presented to you with the aim to condemn. Names of officials, teachers and schools will not be disclosed. My sole purpose is to show there is a pressing need for greater awareness. Even though it was a rough and rocky road for our family up until four years ago, I feel empathy for the educators who were clearly unprepared to deal with children who stutter. Their reaction to my son's speech difficulty was in keeping with the unavailability of information on stuttering in their schools.

Whether a child stutters or not, when he wants to quit school at age 9, something isn't right. All Lucas wanted to do was stay home; he was fixed on the idea that he could not ever do well at school, and trying to break into a large group of friends was impossible. No one wanted to hang around with the kid who couldn't talk. Even though I reminded him that one good friend who really cares about you is all anyone would need, he spent a lot of time trying to come up with better ways to infiltrate the *in* crowd. This only resulted in more feelings of inadequacy because he was convinced that the only thing standing in the way of his making new friends was his stutter.

In following my son's education process very closely, I noted several similarities between today's elementary school programs, and the one I was involved in many years ago. Surely, you can remember the memory work, the recitals, the oral presentation of book reports, the importance of raising your hand and volunteering an answer, the show-and-tell sessions, and those speeches most of us had to prepare at the beginning of each school year to inform our new classmates about all the fun things we did over the summer holidays.

Although I never had any problems expressing myself in front of a group, I recall that many of my classmates dreaded the experience. One friend in particular would always be ill on the day her turn was sure to come up, and she didn't stutter!

As a child, and later on as a teen, I often wondered why my teachers seemed so interested in finding out what I had done over the summer. Was this the process through which they determined who were their better students, or was it simply an opportunity to get to know us on a more personal basis? Regardless of how I felt about this particular teaching approach, it's clear that in our current learning environment, the emphasis remains on effective verbal communication, and if a child who stutters is to succeed, his ability to maintain an acceptable level of fluent speech will be instrumental in getting him through both the elementary and secondary school years.

One might argue that with the advent of the computer, the emphasis has now shifted from verbal communication to communication on internets or other networks. Although I must admit that I have thought of purchasing a portable computer for Lucas to carry around with him at school, I knew that doing so would probably result in his avoiding speech altogether.

The article I wrote gave me a lot of satisfaction, and it forced me to address a lot of mixed feelings I had about my son's stuttering. In fact, it was therapeutic for me. Although Lucas was impressed with some of the story's passages, he never did read it in its entirety. For many reasons, I felt it would have been inappropriate. What I really wanted him to understand was that I was willing to help him go beyond the stutter and the problems it brought on, and I think I was successful at doing just that.

*   *   *

To Lucas, I know how you feel . . . Lucas has a handicap, he stutters. When I first noticed the impediment in his speech, he was just three years old. I was making a tape recording of the children to send to my parents, who were in Florida at the time. I had taken to recording most of the activities I did with the children without their knowledge. It made things easier for everybody, not to mention that the children's chatter was more spontaneous.

The bathtub play time period was being secretly recorded when Lucas and Jonathan, his older brother, began to argue over a toy; one of them would always want what the other one was playing with. Jonathan grabbed the plastic sailboat from Lucas who started screaming, "d-d-d-d-don't, g-g-g-g-give it to me!" Then there was the usual "no, it's mine" response from Jonathan before I could ask Lucas to repeat what he had just said. "Tell him to give me my boat back!" I recall him saying without a stutter, but the previous staccato sounds had already given me cause to worry. I vowed to be on the alert from then on.

I reported this particular incident, and the many subsequent others, to his paediatrician. The intermittent speech dysfluency made it difficult for his doctor to identify the disorder, but by the time he was four, he was attending speech therapy sessions at the Children's Hospital of Eastern Ontario, on a twice-weekly basis. As a concerned parent, I wanted to find the best possible care for him in spite of his young age. I thought if I dealt with the problem right away, he would stand a better chance.

This may sound crazy, but I've often wished he were in a wheelchair instead, *thinking* his life would be far less complicated. His stuttering happens to be a communication disorder, which, unfortunately, has not yet been acknowledged by many in the medical and teaching professions.

Lucas' problem is **not** psychological, as some have implied. Nor is it a disorder which I have personally inflicted on him because I'm a divorced mom. His stutter had surfaced a year prior to my change of residence from the matrimonial home to one of my own, and was not considered severe until many years later. It's true that the first years after my separation were not easy ones for me and my boys, but it didn't mean that I loved my children any less. Thankfully, we did pull through. In fact, I can attribute a large part of my success in overcoming a difficult marital break-up to the love Jonathan, Lucas and I shared.

As later explained to me by fluency specialists,[1] what actually causes stuttering is not clear. Demon possession was once thought to be the cause. In the 1920s and 30s, it was linked to lefthanded children being forced to use their right hands. Then 2000 years of *physiological* theorizing were lost in the 1940s and 50s because of the *psychological* assumption that it was the parents' fault. During this decade, it was assumed that parents were overreacting to children having normal problems in expressing themselves. It was regarded as being a neurotic disorder, or caused by nervousness. But now the pendulum has swung again to the *physiological*.

Because stuttering can run in families,[2] heredity has been noted. And researchers disagree as to why male stutterers outnumber female stutterers by a four-to-one ratio. The most commonly held theory is that males develop language at a slower rate than females, making them more susceptible to inheriting speech disorders.

Both my boys were taught to speak French from the time they were babies. I was of the opinion that making French their mother-tongue would help them get a better job someday. I suppose my growing up as a Francophone in a government city where bilingualism is so important, had a lot to do with it. Their biological father being English-speaking, I knew they would become fluent in both languages in no time at all. In fact, I was hoping that they would learn to speak English much sooner than I had.

When he first started school, Lucas was, like Jonathan, more fluent in French than in English and was enroled in a French program. With the exception of Grade 3, Lucas had to fight for acceptance from Nursery School to Grade 5. It was difficult for his teachers to adapt to his handicap as they had little or no knowledge of the techniques to be used in the classroom. Not only could these techniques have helped the teachers manage his stutter outside the clinical environment, they would have encouraged Lucas to take part in more oral activities.

Year after year, new teachers asked me the same questions over and over again. The first question, of course, was always: "Are you aware that your child has a problem speaking?" and the obvious second question (my all-time favourite) was: "Have you tried getting him the proper care?" There were times when I felt like putting on a look of complete surprise, and pretending I knew nothing about the stuttering. However tempted, I could never go through with it, but I'm sure their reaction would have been amusing for me to watch.

Needless to say, Lucas and I have shared many laughs over the years. There was a need to find the humour in some of the unusual circumstances we experienced because of his stutter. Don't get me wrong, there were plenty of times when we cried, but some situations were so sad, hopeless, and at times, almost ridiculous, we just had to laugh.

Comments about his performance in class were almost always negative. My son hated school, and I couldn't really blame him. Given that there are no special schools for children who stutter, the dysfluent child has no alternative but to try and survive in a world where others have no problem in expressing themselves, and in achieving their goals. Inevitably, my son has been constantly reminded of his inability to be as good as the others in just about any activity. As far as he was concerned, it would have been foolish of him even to try.

Thank goodness for speech class as it gave him a better perspective as to what an enjoyable learning environment should be all about. The bond which had begun to develop between Lucas and his personal speech-language pathologist did wonders for his self-esteem. He needed to hear he was a good kid from someone else besides me.

Just as his clinician did with him to help boost his self-image, rarely did I miss an opportunity to show Lucas how important he is to himself, above all, and to his family. I constantly reminded him to hang on to all of his inner qualities as he did have a lot to offer. Also, when he brought home good test results and a nice note from the teacher (he did get the odd one), it was posted on the fridge door for everyone to see.

Pre-kindergarten and kindergarten were unhappy years for Lucas, although he did like to play with the other children. Looking back on this now, perhaps I could have made things easier for him had I better prepared him for an environment where every other child would speak in a more fluent pattern and at a much quicker rate.

He had the same teacher for both these school years, and I had very little contact with her. As well, the teacher had no contact at all with his speech therapist from the Children's Hospital of Eastern Ontario, who unsuccessfully tried to establish a rapport with her on more than one occasion. At the end of my son's second year with her, I remember her telling me how rarely he ever spoke in her class. I suppose I should have asked her why she waited so long to tell me. I assumed that she was the education specialist and that she had devised other methods through which to assess his performance.

Grade 1 was pretty much the same. At the time, we had been on a waiting list for almost two years before a speech therapist from the Regional Health Care Unit started to visit him at school. These weekly half-hour visits from the speech-language therapist started when he had reached Grade 1. What a relief after two years of leaving work, twice a week, picking him up at school, going to therapy at the hospital, returning him to school and getting myself back to work; I thought this treatment program was great. At least with the therapist going to him, he didn't have to miss as much school.

This new therapist reported it was hard to set up a meeting with the teacher. One would think there would have been some interest shown in what Lucas was doing in therapy. It was not to be. His progress in the classroom was never satisfactory according to this teacher, and our frequent meetings seemed but opportunities for her to signal her displeasure with my child's performance. And this, she did in front of him. Whether Lucas wanted to or not, she told me that she was going to mold him into someone I would be proud of before the year was through.

What she didn't know was that I was already very proud of my son's accomplishments; I knew he was doing the best he could in spite of the school's inability to relate to his stutter.

If Lucas was asked which school year has been the most horrible, there would be no contest it would be Grade 2. He could do nothing right it seemed. As he was then in his fourth year of school, and there was still no hope of a favourable progress report from the teachers, I was beginning to think he was lacking in another area. The administration of the school was not willing to provide me with any assistance, but after several months of telephone calls and through other external contacts, I was successful at getting Lucas assessed by the school's psychologist. I wanted this specialist to find out why my son was not able to meet any of his teacher's requirements when he did so well at speech class and at home.

The results from the psychologist's assessment revealed that my son had better than average capabilities, and in a subsequent meeting I had with him, he indicated there were no obvious reasons why he could not do as well as the others. He mentioned he would visit the classroom from time to time to help smooth things over for Lucas and his teacher. Again, this teacher had little, if any, contact with the speech therapist. Many times, she pointed out to me that she had all the tools at her disposal to teach him and didn't need anybody's help. I wasn't suggesting she needed help to teach, I was merely recommending a telephone call or a brief meeting with Lucas' speech therapist so she could get to know my son better.

Things did not improve. In fact, they got much worse especially after the psychologist started dropping in unannounced on Lucas' teacher. She did not appreciate the intrusions. I'm sure she viewed his visits as a threat, which probably made her dislike Lucas, and his terrible mother, even more.

At one point, she was so uptight about the psychologist's involvement that she started screaming at me one afternoon when I went to pick up Lucas at school. She warned me to stop meddling in her affairs, and if I didn't think she was good enough for my son, perhaps I should remove him from her class altogether. She got so red in the face, I feared she would have a stroke. I took Lucas by the hand, and said, very quietly, that we would be back after she had had time to cool off. She kept on screaming and waving her arms in anger as we walked quickly down the hall to the stairs. My insides were shaking by the time we finally made it outside; it was a troubling experience for me, and I wondered what kind of an effect all this was having on Lucas.

I started by apologizing to him for getting the psychologist involved, and I assured him all I was trying to do was make things better for him at school. He was way ahead of me. "Don't be scared Mom, she does that to me all the time!" It struck me that even at his young age, my child was so resilient, it was almost frightening. If my Grade 2 teacher had yelled at my mom and me like that, I would have cried for a week, and my mother would never have set foot in any school again. She would have sent my Dad!

I kept Lucas from school the next day. The principal called to offer her apologies for her teacher's outburst. She regretted the teacher's unprofessional conduct and added she would be on an indefinite leave of absence. She mumbled something about a "burn-out". I didn't dare mention that I had already noted the teacher's tired demeanour and impatient tone at the *Meet the Teacher Night* back in mid-October. I don't think this principal thought that I, as a parent, was supposed to be that perceptive. She asked if I would consider bringing Lucas back as a new teacher had already been assigned to his class for the next few weeks. The regular teacher did not return to work until the end of the year.

[It was during this year that there was another change in our family. Having lived on my own for over three years, my boys and I decided it was time to build a new life for us. Despite the numerous times Jonathan would take it upon himself to introduce his mom to perfect strangers living in our apartment building, I decided to give in to my feelings for a man I already knew and had met on my own. It wasn't until we moved into our new home together that Jonathan, Lucas and I realized how much we really needed someone like Paul.]

To date, Lucas' best school year was Grade 3. His new teacher made up for the Grade 2 teacher in spades! She took the time to discuss his progress with his speech therapist on a continuous basis, from the beginning of the year right up to the end. She even invited the speech therapist to come speak to her class to explain what stuttering was all about, and to make his classmates understand the special efforts constantly required of an individual who lives with this problem.

Consequently, Lucas had a terrific year. There were a couple of times when he did slip up, but this teacher's great interpersonal skills made it easy to discuss both the good and the not-so-good situations. After all, not all children can be on their best behaviour at all times. In that regard, Lucas could be as mischievous as the next kid. However, the support and encouragement he received from his Grade 3 teacher had a tremendous impact on his oral and overall performance.

These days, when times get complicated, I often find myself longing for the kind words Lucas' Grade 3 teacher often spoke to me. It felt so nice to hear my son had a great week, not to mention that it made my going to work that year far less stressful. To this day, Lucas speaks of this teacher with great admiration. He realizes how fortunate he was to have had her. I was grateful for the impact she had on his developing an interest to learn.

In Grade 4, Lucas had to change schools as we moved into a new neighbourhood. Remembering how threatened teachers from his other school had felt whenever I suggested they discuss my son's handicap with his speech therapist, this time, I thought perhaps the best approach would be to take a back seat and let the education specialists cope with my son's severe stutter on their own. I don't know of other mothers who have had to report to schools on as many occasions as I have.

My colleagues have always wondered why teachers were calling me so frequently at work, when the only times they ever had to get involved was to pick up a report card or attend a school play. Although my career has always been secondary to my responsibilities as a mother, I've often been made to feel that I shouldn't be involved in anything else but Lucas' speech-related problematic episodes at school. In view of my youngest son's situation, trying to pay as much attention to Jonathan has never been easy. I've always been thankful for his self-sufficient nature which helped to ease my guilt on more than one occasion.

Even though Lucas was then beginning to show signs of fear and frustration, he did learn from his Grade 4 teacher. The times we met, I found her to be pleasant and genuinely concerned about his speech problem. His marks were relatively good. It was around that time, however, that Lucas cancelled his speech therapy service. I wasn't aware of the fact that he was then beginning to feel more and more embarrassed about his stuttering, and having the therapist come to his class and whisk him away for a session only added to his predicament. I couldn't believe he would deprive himself of her visits when I knew his speech class was essentially the only thing he liked about school.

Neither did I know he had become the butt of jokes for many children. How cruel. The therapist reported there wasn't much point in forcing him to come to therapy if he no longer wanted to work at it. Too many others needed the service. There aren't enough speech therapists working for our Regional Health Unit of Eastern Ontario, so their time cannot be wasted. It was probably best to let him be; should he want to start up again, his speech therapist advised she would be there for him.

As a result, his speech began to deteriorate to the point where it was hard to understand him, and I noticed several other changes in him. He was becoming an expert at finding ways to avoid speech altogether. For example, he had learned to make such good use of his hands to communicate that except for the odd grunt or nod, there was hardly any need for him to talk.

I let the summer go by, and tried to ignore the twitches and the *hicuppy* sounds, and we concentrated on doing fun things instead. Aren't children supposed to do that? Up until then, my son had to make up for so much school work, in addition to his speech therapy assignments, there never was much time left for anything else. Camping on the shore of Lake Ontario turned out to be an enjoyable and relaxing holiday for everyone.

And so, Lucas reached Grade 5. If anyone was to ask me which school year has been the most difficult, I'd say this was the one. I don't know if it's because I was more aware of my child's unhappiness at school, a situation which had become alarming in that I feared it would never get any better. What was going to happen to him if cooperation could not be obtained from the teachers? I must admit, I did not blame his Grade 5 teacher entirely, as she certainly was not prepared for her year with a child who stutters. Nevertheless, there are a lot of things she could have done differently.

Although school problems remained the same, we made some progress with my son's speech therapy. In the fall of 1989, following up on a article which appeared in our local newspaper, I contacted the Head of the Stuttering Therapy Program at the Rehabilitation Centre of the Royal Ottawa Health Care Group. Shortly after, Lucas began treatment sessions with Marie Poulos, who became his new speech-language pathologist, a great friend and confidante. Marie made an exception for Lucas because at the time, the Precision Fluency Shaping Program (PFSP) was offered to adults and to some adolescents in their late teens.

Later on, I learned that similar programs were available in just three locations in Canada: Ottawa and Toronto in Ontario and Edmonton, Alberta. Lucas did well and I was particularly impressed with the Ottawa program which was more intensive in comparison to all the other treatment opportunities in which he had been involved in the past. The best thing about the program was that he loved to go. The many adults involved in his therapy all showed him the support and the love he needed to overcome his handicap and to come out of his shell. If only his school could have worked hand in hand with some of these people, his education environment could have been less stressful for him.

The poor progress reports from September 1989 to January 1990, the many telephone calls during my working day, the notes from the teacher indicating that Lucas would not cooperate in any activity, especially oral ones, convinced me to request a meeting with the principal and the Grade 5 teacher. It was time, once again, to intervene on Lucas' behalf.

At this meeting, I tried to explain that my son would not likely ever be fluent and he wasn't stuttering to annoy anyone; it was just his unique way of voicing sounds. I pointed out to them that he functioned very well elsewhere, and that I suspected the serious problems they were reporting were probably speech-related.

As his troubles always seemed to be triggered at recess and noon breaks, I asked them if they knew of the continuous amount of teasing he was subjected to. They didn't. Surely, they could understand that to be constantly laughed at by his peers was not conducive to a refreshed and relaxed frame of mind upon a return to the classroom. The teasing made his blood boil. He would become very angry and even more frustrated with his speech knowing he couldn't even report these incidents to any of the school's authorities.

I asked if they were aware of my child's battle with his tongue, his lips, his teeth, and his ability to inhale the right amount of air in his lungs to produce **a single stretched sound** which may, or may not be clearly understood. They were not. We had reached January, and yet no request for my child's speech therapy file from the Children's Hospital had even been made. At the time of registration in September of 1988, however, I had provided them with the name of his therapist and had also granted them permission to request my son's speech dossier.

I explained that school was becoming more and more confusing for Lucas. His speech therapist showed him how to make different sounds so he could control his stutter while voicing the words. He was congratulated for the effort he put into his therapy, but at school, he was told to start over again because his teacher said he was not pronouncing his words properly. He often told me he didn't know what to do any more.

To show that my son's life clearly revolved around his speech, I reported the following situation to the principal and his teacher. Prior to Christmas, I had helped Lucas with one of his school projects. He got a lot of enjoyment from working on this particular assignment, but he seemed reluctant to hand it in. In questioning his reasons, I found out that the project was an oral presentation. I knew then why he had insisted on keeping his sentences so short.

In order to encourage him, I told him he would not be expected to present orally because I would call his teacher and explain his fear of talking in front of kids who laugh at him. I told him I would ask that he be allowed to do his presentation at recess, when no one else would be around to hear him, or perhaps he could be allowed to present in front of a few of his close friends who didn't find his stuttering amusing.

As it turned out, his teacher either forgot about my telephone call or did not feel that Lucas should be given special treatment and he had to present in front of the entire class. When he came home that evening, he was genuinely upset with me for having lied to him. He felt I had tricked him into being further exposed as a "dummy" (as he used to say) in an area in which everybody else was so much better than he. I thought I had selected an excellent example to show how his stutter played a major role in his life and to adequately demonstrate the importance of getting the school, speech-language pathologist and parent to work together. It wasn't working.

Finally, I suggested they get in touch with his speech therapist who would be happy to come to the school and make a presentation to the Grade 5 students and their teacher. It took from January to mid-March to arrange the visit, as the school officials and the concerned teacher remained unconvinced that this would be helpful to Lucas. When it finally came about, the students and the teacher were very receptive to the information presented by Marie and two of her colleagues.

Another matter I brought up at a subsequent meeting with officials at the school was the production of a film in which Lucas had been asked to take part. At the request of a Toronto, Ontario, film producer, I asked the principal if he would agree to let a camera crew into the school. This film was being produced in an effort to better inform our Canadian school system in the area of stuttering. Sponsorship had already been obtained from several organizations who viewed this idea with enthusiasm. The principal replied that he would have to do a lot of serious thinking on this one. I wondered why, but not wanting to jeopardize the project altogether, I thought I would give him the time he needed to decide on his school's involvement in the film.

The following week, I contacted two other principals from different school boards to ask what their reaction would be to such an opportunity if my son was in attendance at one of their schools. Both felt that the film project was an exceptionally good idea. They added that the request would undoubtedly have to be channelled properly, but because so little is known about stuttering, they added that it was an initiative worth undertaking.

Even after the Toronto producer travelled to Ottawa to meet with the principal on two separate occasions, he was not willing to involve his school in the film. When I spoke to him a week later, his reply was he still needed time to discuss it with his staff and superiors, but added he was fearful of negative consequences should he decide to open his doors to a camera crew. I failed to understand the logic behind his response as I felt this film would be an excellent teaching aid. My son's classmates could have benefitted from such an experience, not to mention that it could have cleared the path for others with communication disorders who would attend this school in years to come. My disappointment could no longer be concealed.

I knew I had a lot of work ahead of me in order to effect a more positive change in how my son was being treated at school. In the mean-time, I told Lucas to hang on to the written message of hope given to him by a dear friend by the name of Jock: *"May your tongue untangle so well that you NEVER stop talking."*

*   *   *

Shortly after I wrote this story, one last incident happened at school. Lucas' regular teacher had to undergo surgery and a supply teacher had taken over the class. The new teacher found my son's stuttering most amusing. He started to mimic him in Porky Pig style which encouraged the rest of his classmates to laugh at him every time he spoke! Finally, Lucas decided he had tolerated this teacher's insensitivity long enough and ran away on a day when his class was on a special field trip.

I was frantic when the principal called to inform me that my son had suddenly disappeared, and somehow I knew this latest situation would also be connected to his speech problem. They were away from the classroom setting, and I thought it would be doubly difficult for the teacher to have any control over what could happen to Lucas during a class outing. It wasn't until later that afternoon that I found out he hadn't been running away from a class bully, but from the teacher him-self! Fortunately, Lucas had had the good sense to hide in the travel bus which would be taking him back to school. When I arrived in the princi-pal's office, Lucas came crashing into me, wrapped his arms around my waist and wouldn't let go. The day had been a really devastating experi-ence for him. I could feel his heart pounding right through me and it was all I could do to restrain myself from physically attacking the teacher and the principal. Instead, I agreed to sit down with Lucas who continued to cling to me while excuses were provided. I listened and I left.

I had already made up my mind to find another school for Lucas. The nightmarish experiences had to stop. I was called to another meeting at the school where one of the school board's superintendents offered further apologies for the actions of the supply teacher, the school principal and Lucas' regular teacher. But too much damage had been done. It was time to move on.

*   *   *

As part of Lucas' speech therapy program, there were scheduled refresher courses which took place over different weekends throughout the year. It was to one of these sessions that Jock Carlisle, author of *Tangled Tongue*, had been invited as guest speaker. Marie Poulos, Lucas' speech-language pathologist, insisted that I join them on that particular Saturday, because she thought Dr. Carlisle could help me with the story I had been writing about Lucas.

Jock was as interesting in person as he was as a writer. His excellent sense of humour and his perfectly candid style of recounting fascinating stories from his past made it exciting to listen. I stayed after his presentation, met his wife Joan, and asked him if he wouldn't mind editing my story, and once he had read it perhaps he would have some advice for me as to where, and to whom I should be sending it. "Oh," he said, "I'd be delighted to edit your story. I love to make red marks all over someone else's copy!" I explained I didn't have a conclusion for my story yet. "What?" he exclaimed, "you want me to edit a story that has no ending!" I told him I would rush home immediately to write it and that it would be in the mail the following day. I met my deadline.

*   *   *

In late March 1990, I received the following letter from Jock.

> Thank you for the revised manuscript. I like the bit at the end about Jock and Lucas, "may his tongue untangle . . . "
>
> You must be sure of your objective. If the story is designed as an effective tool to influence school boards, politicians, teachers, etc. it is too long. The shorter version should grab them.
>
> Your story is well written and obviously comes from the heart. Unfortunately, for the audience you are aiming it at, it will have a low impact. I suggest you write a high impact, effective summary of not more than one or two pages. Pick out the key points in your story and sock it to them. Then add the rest as an appendix for further reading.
>
> Incidentally, why not write a letter to the Minister of Education for Ontario, and include a copy of your story as an appendix, or try your own local Member of Parliament. One point to mention to you, if you take this problem higher, Lucas may get some of the backlash at school. I think the risk is worth it, but Lucas may not.
>
> Lucas will encounter pain and frustration. Coping with those can be learned. Above all, try to get him to take consistent therapy. If his peers jeer at him for being different, he must learn to ignore them for the minijerks they are. He will find friends, as valuable as jewels, true friends who will support him and help in his battles. You cannot spare him the tough path, the very tough path, but you can, with the therapist's help, teach him how to traverse that path and deal with the monsters he meets on the way and keep his self-respect.
>
> Lucas is a great guy, just starting on the tough path we all trod. At his age, it can either crush him or make him into something very worthwhile, someone who has been through the fire and come out with a steel will forged within him. He is somebody special; never let him forget that. Later he can learn to help himself by helping others.
>
> All the best to yourself and Lucas. Thank goodness he has a caring parent.
>
> Jock Carlisle
Paid-up Member of the Clan of the Tangled Tongue

Once I got the go-ahead from Lucas, I took Jock's advice and wrote a high-impact letter to the Minister of Education for Ontario. In his July 27, 1990, response, the Honourable Sean Conway stated:

I understand your being discouraged by the lack of understanding by individual teachers about Lucas' stuttering, and your disappointment with the lack of approval for the school's involvement in the film about stuttering. The film appears to be a worthwhile endeavour which will, as you have indicated, provide a vehicle for promoting greater awareness for stuttering. You are no doubt encouraged by the fact that it will be produced, despite the difficulties, and will therefore be available for use in the educational community.

You may wish to continue to communicate with staff in the Eastern Ontario Regional Office of the Ministry of Education who will be able to assist you in making information about the availability of the film accessible to school boards.

I am particularly pleased to learn from ministry staff that you are satisfied that your son's needs are being met more appropriately at this time.

Sean Conway
Minister of Education for Ontario

*   *   *

I wondered how, but the Minister's regional office had already informed him that I had found a new school for Lucas in late April 1990.

Notes

1. Czulinski, Winnie. 1992. *Stuttering: You Living With Verve.* June 1992 Edition. Pages 30-31.
2. Sutter, Paul J. 1994. *In a Manner of Speaking: Strategies for Stutterers.* Today's Parent. November 1994 Edition. Pages 102-103 and 104.

CHAPTER 3

DISCOVERING THAT STUTTERING IS NOTHING TO BE ASHAMED OF

After two weeks of well-deserved holidays for mother and son, we found another school in late April 1990. I had been encouraged by friends and a school board trustee to try another school board altogether.

Things were actually looking up (for the first few weeks anyway); Lucas was adapting well and his new teacher had nothing but good things to report. I couldn't help but be taken aback when in early June, the principal asked that I meet with him at the school. He had something important to discuss, and preferred not to get into it over the phone. It was at this meeting I was informed that Lucas would have to repeat his year. According to the principal and his new teacher, my son was so far behind he wouldn't be able to cope with the Grade 6 program. Looking back on this now, I realize, of course, I should never have agreed to have my son repeat his year, especially when measures to have a pedagogical assessment had not been taken. I honestly believed, at the time, that the new school had his best interests at heart.

The principal insisted I tell Lucas immediately. He was called out from class, and together we walked to the play structure area in the school yard where I told him the bad news. He was crushed and so was I. We sat in the sandbox and we cried. He, because he knew the pain and the challenge of having to start anew with classmates and teachers who have never been exposed to his stuttering, and I, because no matter how gently I broke the news to him, I was still telling him he wasn't as good as the fluent kids – when I'd been stressing the exact opposite since he was old enough to understand me. Such tough times for a 9 year old, I thought. It just didn't seem fair.

I had just completed a long search to find this second French school in April, but I told Lucas I would be willing to find him another if he wanted to start somewhere else, where no one would know he was repeating his year. He thought about it for a few days, and decided it would be easier to go back to the same school in September seeing they already knew about his stuttering. Another reason why he wanted to go back was that he was also guaranteed at least one friend. The son of one of our neighbours also attended this school, and they would be in the same class.

He would be 10 on July 5, and in view of everything that had happened, I thought of doing something extra special for Lucas to help him put the past behind him. His speech-language pathologist had told me about the San Francisco-based organization called the *National Stuttering Project (NSP)*, and the annual conventions it held for people who stutter. Parts of this second story were written as we travelled back to Canada from Anaheim, California, where we had attended our first conference on stuttering.

*   *   *

Lucas goes to L.A. . . . It had been pointed out to me that taking Lucas to an NSP conference would enable us to visualize just how warm, loving and crazy people can be. So we quickly packed our bags as we were both anxious to experience an event which turned out to be more than just a special trip – it was a revelation.

Having arrived a couple of days prior to the conference, we had some free time to do all the *touristy* things. Naturally, Disneyland was first on our agenda. All we had to do was cross the parking lot of our hotel, and there we were at the main gate. In spite of the record high temperature of 114 degrees, we were able to take in all of the major attractions, including the *Star Wars Tour* in *Tomorrowland* and the *Dick Tracy Musical Review*. Lucas was delighted. He was in such high spirits that once in a line-up to purchase whatever could quench our thirst, he said he was going to ask for his own drink. I wondered if he was under some kind of Magical Kingdom spell. Normally, I would have spared him the agony, but I thought it best to let him fly like an eagle and do his own thing. It was a disaster. But he survived, and his Sprite on ice tasted like no other did before.

Our one-day round trip to Universal Studios was equally exciting. Although the temperature went up to 116, nothing could stop us from visiting as many sites as possible. We saw *Mr. T's* van, the *Miami Vice Stunt Team*, the movie sets of *Conan the Barbarian, ET, Back to the Future, Psycho* and *Jaws*. I heard nothing but "Hey Mommy, look at this!" for six straight hours.

On our third day in California, the conference began. I enjoyed the Carl Dell presentation on the opening day. Dr. Dell is a senior speech-language pathologist who runs a successful clinic at Eastern Illinois University. I found his style both captivating and informative. With commendable control, he spoke of the fear of ordering food, using the telephone, or speaking in front of a large group of people. His approach was humorous at times, with a realistic twist intended to inspire his listeners.

The open-mike sessions were great too. I, as a fluent person, wouldn't dream of speaking in front of a packed ballroom! It was bad enough that I found myself stammering, trying to find my words in English the whole time I was there. This sort of thing often happens to me when I find myself in a completely English environment where I can't revert to French to save my skin. Speaking in front of small groups is fine, but large audiences are too hard on the system (mine anyway). Written words are for me the best vehicle to voice my thoughts and feelings. I leave public speech to people who stutter. After what I witnessed at these sessions, they certainly have a better handle on it than I ever could.

A friend by the name of Tania took care of Lucas for me while I attended a workshop by Janice Westbrook, Ph.D., a speech-language pathologist from Texas. To this day, I believe it was Janice's presentation which made me come to grips with our personal situation. She proceeded to greet everyone, and then she asked parents in the audience to tell her how their children's stutter made them feel. She got a lot of appropriate responses; some said it made them feel sad, guilty, helpless, discouraged . . . all the normal feelings.

Then Janice said the responses we had given her were good, but asked if there wasn't something we had forgotten. As no one could come up with anything else, she asked us to think about this one: "Doesn't watching your child stutter drive you crazy at times?" The room fell silent for a few moments. Then, there was laughter in the room as many of us realized that this woman had just voiced what we sometimes felt, but being the good parents that we were, we would never dream of being vocal about such a feeling. So there I sat . . . my secret was out, and it felt good. Yes, there were times when I found my son's stuttering hard to take, but it didn't mean I was a bad mother.

Janice Westbrook told us it was OK to have such feelings; we wouldn't be normal if we didn't admit to them. Facing my own emotions and fears about my son's stuttering was the key to helping him live with this difficulty. I vowed to stop looking for cures or quick *fixes*, and wanted to do my best to encourage him to make use of his speech techniques. One could say that Janice had been successful at recharging the batteries of many parents, including mine.

Thanks to Al Utronki, one of Lucas good friends from his treatment centre in Ottawa, John Ahlbach, Executive Director of the NSP, and Des Mahoney, a golf pro from Hawaii, the highlight of Lucas' trip was a meeting with Dave Taylor of the L.A. Kings. He got to spend some private time with Dave and his wife Beth. His autograph book came in handy. Following the Dave Taylor presentation (which I might add created quite an impact on the little one), Lucas was asked to present his hockey hero with a plaque. I couldn't have been more proud.

We were both looking forward to coming home. It seemed that I had so much to write about, countless ideas to pursue, and Lucas did even better: he came home with a Dave Taylor hockey stick. (The Dave Taylor hockey stick was given to me by Mike Healey, a gentleman from Petaluma, California, who bid $300.00 for the stick at the auction which followed the banquet dinner. I was moved by his kind and generous gesture.)

While we maintained our economy class seats, this stick travelled first class, in a compartment which met with the approval of its proud new owner. He had no problem expressing his concerns in this particular regard! And besides, he couldn't afford to let anything happen to his treasure: he was contemplating charging an admission fee to his bedroom wall of fame. Unfortunately for him, it was my duty as a mother to put a damper on his get-rich-quick scheme: "Free admission," I said, "even for your brother."

*   *   *

The trip to Anaheim certainly did wonders for Lucas. (The MasterCard people were equally pleased with the charges I made during that week.) More importantly, the trip gave him all the incentive he needed to do well throughout his three-week intensive therapy program, the Precision Fluency Shaping Program (PFSP) which began in early July 1990. He had been preparing for this special treatment opportunity since January with his personal speech-language pathologist, Marie Poulos. The weekly therapy sessions he had with her were a lead-in to the adult-oriented program. Lucas knew how lucky he was to take part in this intensive program and he was determined to succeed.

In comparison to the weekly speech therapy sessions, various intensive programs are highly successful treatment opportunities for people who stutter. In recent years, I have talked to many speech-language pathologists working for various school boards or involved in the Home Care Program offered by our Regional Health Unit. They all agreed that intensive programs are probably the best way to treat stuttering. Most found that trying to treat stuttering through 30-minute weekly or bi-weekly sessions can become frustrating for both the therapist and the child because it takes so long to make progress. Consequently, some children give up on their therapy altogether. The speech therapy programs currently offered to school-aged children by school board specialists on occasion or by speech-language pathologists working for the Regional Health Unit, are essentially maintenance exercises which would be more effective if a child had previously undergone an intensive program.

I came across a written assignment Lucas had completed during his PFSP. It shows he had learned that success can only be achieved through a lot of hard work.

Speech Reconstruction for People who Stutter
by Lucas

The STRETCHED SYLLABLE target is when you stretch your letters. To proceed with this technique you must slow your speech down and try to keep it calm. It will take a lot of practice and patience, but it's worth it. You really get to control your speech instead of it controlling you.

The first sound should be held for one full second. The whole word will take two seconds, but you must use your stopwatch until you get to the point you know when it is two seconds. But there is a lot more to do before you get to that point. You must get used to using the stopwatch first. It is not that easy at first, but the more you practice, the better your speech gets. You have to practice as much as you can.

There are letters you cannot stretch. Those are *h, f, ch, s, sh,* and the voiceless *th.* All these letters are Class III sounds. The vowels like *a, e, i, o, u* are Class I sounds you can stretch.

Why do you stutter? There are so many reasons, you wouldn't believe it. Some actually are not true, like when we were born and didn't get enough air. Wrong. Even I don't know for sure if that's true. I think people who stutter have different vocal folds. That's my theory.

*   *   *

Parents and friends were invited to the graduation ceremony. Lucas graduated with top honours and the smile on his face said it all.

To show the significant progress Lucas made with his speech after his participation in the intensive therapy program, I will use excerpts from the initial **Assessment Report** and the subsequent **Progress Summary** which were both prepared by Marie Poulos. Copies of these reports were given to me by Marie for personal delivery to Lucas' teachers at the beginning of each school year. She wanted his teachers and other school officials to be informed about his speech difficulty and of his progress with therapy. She had also hoped that upon receipt of these reports, the educators directly involved with Lucas' schooling would establish some form of contact with her.

Assessment Report, November 1989

Lucas was seen for assessment of stuttering behaviour on November 15, 1989. His mother reports that Lucas, who is now in Grade 5, speaks spontaneously (meaning without making use of speech techniques) in class even though he is familiar with and can use fluency skills well. He does not like being called out of class for therapy and has requested to receive treatment outside of school.

The stutter is characterized by multiple sound and syllable repetitions, prolongations and sound blockages. Secondary features include head jerking, eye close, body tapping and tension noted in the facial musculature as he tries to release himself from a block. Management of breath stream is poor as he frequently tries to speak on residual air. The stutter significantly impedes communication. Lucas stutters on approximately 33% of syllables spoken in conversation and 40% of syllables read.

Lucas' stutter is present every day but is situationally variable. He stutters more in situations in which he is anxious about his speech. He reports the severity of his stutter is about the same when he speaks in English or in French.

He is aware of the variability of his stutter and is now beginning to avoid or hold back in speaking situations. He talked openly about his stutter throughout the assessment. He understands that carry over of fluency requires practice and use of the fluency skills in every day speaking situations.

Lucas presents with a moderate to severe stutter which significantly interferes with the efficiency of his day-to-day communication. It is recommended that he begin individual therapy sessions on a weekly basis beginning in January of 1990 and follow this with his participation in an intensive stuttering treatment program scheduled for the summer of the same year.

Progress Summary, July 1990

Lucas participated in the intensive stuttering treatment program scheduled between July 3 and July 26, 1990, at the Rehabilitation Centre in Ottawa, Ontario.

He learned the fluency skills associated with the PFSP. He learned all targets with ease and could achieve skills well in structured practice activities within the clinic.

He engaged in the following transfer activities: shopping plaza visits, telephone calls, formal speeches and conversations with strangers. He required considerable external prompting to use his targets in all of these situations. When attempting to use fluency skills, he demonstrated slight difficulty initiating speech. This usually resulted from his difficulty achieving the full breath and gentle onset targets. At times, starter mechanics such as "well," "but," etc. were used. Once speech was initiated, however, Lucas was able to maintain reasonable control of his speech using his fluency skills. Upon completion of the program, he could maintain reasonable control of his speech in a variety of speaking contexts.

Percentage of dysfluency:
Pre program: 18.1 %
Post program: 7.5%

Rate of speech:
Pre program: 71.5 syllables per minute
Post program: 174 syllables per minute

Confidence to enter speaking situations:
Pre program: 48.5%
Post program: 99.52%

Confidence to use slow normal speech:
Post program: 97.85%

Lucas made considerable gains in fluency and in his confidence to enter social speaking situations. It is questionable, however, whether he is mature enough to maintain these gains. It was felt reasonable for Lucas to maintain some degree of target use both at home and in the school. Lucas will continue to be followed at this centre for maintenance therapy.

It's important to know that after a child or an adult who stutters undergoes a treatment program, there is always the possibility of a relapse. Although my son had acquired the skills to control his stutter, maintenance therapy was required to help him retain his current level of speech. He has been seen on a monthly basis since the completion of his intensive program. When away from the clinical environment, however, it was easy to slip back into the old speech patterns. I noticed that the precision and accuracy of his skills deteriorated slightly, which led to a reduction in his fluency control. With prompting, he could usually get himself back on track, but under conditions of high pressure, speech control was limited.

In the classroom, this meant that control would be variable when reading aloud or when answering questions. His speech would not always be fluent and there would be some struggle and tension. More stressful speaking events, such as making an oral presentation, would bring about greater speaking anxiety which, in turn, would also interfere with speech control. Suggestions were also prepared by Marie Poulos for distribution to Lucas' new teachers in the hope they would implement the necessary remedial strategies to help him achieve and maintain fluency when at school. *(Tips on* **How to help the student who stutters** *are included in Chapter Seven.)*

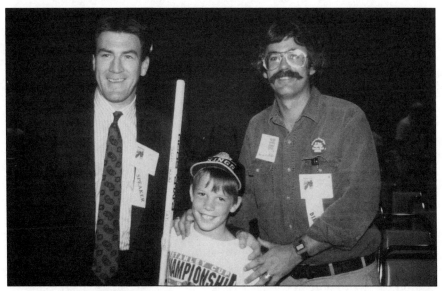

Lucas with Dave Taylor and another good friend, John Ahlbach, Executive Director of the National Stuttering Project (NSP)

CHAPTER 4

MORE PROBLEMS AT SCHOOL

As agreed in June 1990, Lucas returned to the same school in September. To help relieve him of some of the anxiety he always felt when school was about to start, I had made arrangements for him to meet with his new teachers and principal at the school in mid-August. Although his meeting with the new Home Room teacher had eased his mind, I could tell that it was going to be difficult for him to start Grade 5 over again with new classmates who were all one year younger. With the exception of two or three close friends who did not find his stutter amusing, Lucas was subjected to more teasing from the rest of the group; one child in particular called him Lu-lu-lu-Lucas from September right through to early May.

There have been times when no matter how hard I tried, it seemed impossible to change the attitudes of certain individuals towards people who stutter. Our experience with this school was another one of those times.

At the August meeting, I provided the administration of the school and the two teachers with documentation on stuttering prepared by American fluency specialists. My son's personal speech-language pathologist, Marie Poulos, thinking that a proactive approach would alleviate some of the unpleasant situations experienced in the past, insisted I give them a short but detailed brochure on how to help the student who stutters.

Also included in that package were the results from Lucas' intensive therapy program and a tape recording of the winning speech he made at the PFSP graduation ceremony. The tape recording was specifically provided to help teachers appreciate his use of new speech techniques, and the considerable effort involved in order to achieve controlled fluency. At the same time, I thought it appropriate to give these officials the name and telephone number of my son's speech-language pathologist.

I remember thanking Marie for the documentation she had prepared for me to deliver to the school, and I also recall asking her if doing so would get me into hot water with the new school which could lead to subsequent repercussions for Lucas. I reminded her that previous teachers had not been receptive to this kind of information. "Nonsense," she said, "you worry too much, and it's time to let your guard down and give these people a chance for Lucas' sake. And besides, schools do not have access to many publications on stuttering, and this brochure will take but a few minutes to read. It's the only way teachers will be able to help themselves to tips on how to cope with your son's stutter," she argued.

A few months later, however, Marie found herself apologizing to Lucas and me for assuming that the new teachers would take the time to read the information she had provided.

One of the main reasons I was sold on this school was the fact that the principal himself was a man who stuttered. One would think we had finally found an educator who could empathize with my child's stuttering problem, but as kids say these days. . . *NOT!* In fact, we were doomed from the start.

As mentioned to me later on by the school board's own speech-language pathologist, Lucas' new principal had never been to speech therapy. And according to him, anyone who suffers from this disorder can overcome it by simply remaining calm at all times, just as he did. Over the months that followed, I observed that his method was not fool-proof.

After having spent most of an afternoon in his principal's office for splashing water on a little girl's pants while playing with his friend at recess, Lucas came home one day and said: "He wants me to stay in his office until I calm down and learn to relax, but if I get more relaxed than I already am, I'm gonna pass out!" That sounded really funny to me, but seeing he was in no mood to laugh, I explained that I understood his frustration and perhaps the best thing to do would be to humour the principal for the time being. I added, naively, there was a possibility that some day, his principal would notice that it takes a lot more than a relaxed body to control a stutter.

Lucas was in his second week of school when the English teacher informed her students on a Friday afternoon that on the following Monday and Tuesday, they would be asked to make an oral presentation on what they had done over the summer. Had the English teacher read the information on stuttering, she would have known to give Lucas a couple of other options instead of having to present orally in front of classmates who had already begun to give him a hard time about his bumpy speech. Inevitably, this meant I had to deal with my son's justified fear of a formal speech for an entire weekend. He cried himself to sleep, cried in his sleep and woke up with a stomach ache three days in a row.

I tried to comfort him as much as I could and, although he hated every minute of it, he did practice his speech about his trip to L.A.. My husband Paul and I convinced him to bring his Dave Taylor hockey stick which would be helpful in diverting the students' attention away from his stutter should his speech break down in mid-sentence. Not only did he bring the stick, but he brought a framed picture of Dave and himself.

On Monday evening, the day before he was to speak, he scribbled his speech on a piece of paper which he wanted to keep in his pocket as he planned to practice at morning recess. On Tuesday, Mother sat on pins and needles all day, hoping she had instilled enough self-confidence in her son over the weekend to help him survive the experience. He did, but there were several complications.

His first stumbling block was not being able to remove his treasured hockey stick from the principal's office when the time came for English class. He had stored his prized possessions there for safe-keeping when he arrived at school in the morning. Unfortunately for him, the principal was called away and the acting administrator wanted an explanation as to why these things were being taken away from his office.

One thing Lucas could always count on was a mechanical failure in his speech when being asked a surprise question by a new authority figure. Instead of explaining why he needed his things, he chose to make a run for the bathroom as he was beginning to feel queasy. Then he managed to muster enough courage to ask the school secretary if he could call home. Hearing his completely erratic speech, it took some time for me to get the whole story.

I asked him to let me speak to the secretary, and the whole matter was resolved in a matter of minutes. I asked her to tell the principal why my son needed his hockey stick and his picture, and would she kindly go and inform the English teacher about the problems Lucas had been having. Then I went over some basic speech therapy exercises with him on the phone to help him regain his confidence. Once we practised the slow-normal rate of speech, and I was able to reassure him he sounded great, he agreed he was feeling less anxious and in better control. When I hung up, I prayed he wouldn't be asked to make another oral presentation for a long while, a very, very long while.

As expected, Lucas' presentation did not go as well as he would have liked, and this was another time when he was upset with me for having cooperated with the school to get him to speak in front of his entire class. As far as he was concerned, he stood a better chance at making new friends if no one suspected that he stuttered. Now that everybody had heard him make a fool of himself, he knew even tougher times were ahead.

Lucas had reason to be concerned. Once again he had become the butt of jokes on a continual basis. I found myself wondering why laughing at a physically-challenged child is considered improper behaviour while making fun of a child's stuttering difficulty continues to be acceptable. When I reported this to Marie, she mentioned that the incidents surrounding Lucas' stutter could have easily been avoided if his teachers had contacted her at the beginning of the year to ask her to come to the school and explain what stuttering was all about. However, neither one of them had done so, and in mid-November, she came up with another plan to help improve Lucas' situation in class.

She gave me a second copy of the National Stuttering Project (NSP) poster which reads *If You Stutter, You're in Good Company* and features famous people who stuttered like Marilyn Monroe, Winston Churchill, Charles Darwin, Lewis Carroll (author of *Alice's Adventures in Wonderland*), King George VI, Isaac Newton, and Aristotle. (The first copy she gave me of this poster still hangs in my home office.) My son was proud to bring this poster to school, a measure viewed by fluency specialists as an excellent means to create greater awareness for stuttering.

The teacher put the poster up, but left the job of discussing this new addition to her class to a supply teacher who obviously didn't know how to approach the topic. Except for one brave little boy and his best friend, the rest of the students broke out into uncontrollable fits of laughter when the poster was introduced to the class. Lucas' speech was seriously affected by this episode, and it seemed like hours before he could tell me all that had happened.

As the supply teacher explained to me later that evening (it took some time for me to go down the list of telephone numbers under his name, but I was determined to make contact) he had moved on to discuss something else as soon as he noticed how humiliating the experience had been for my son, but he admitted that it took a long time before he could regain control of the class.

In late March, one of the teachers called my home to report that Lucas was being disruptive in her class. She explained that she couldn't understand why he was acting this way because he had been such a good student. I told her that I too was having great difficulty understanding what was happening with Lucas when all I heard at home was how much he liked his English class and the exciting Gordon Korman book he had been reading as one of his class assignments.

In an effort to get to the root of the problem, I asked her several other questions about my son's recent behaviour. She volunteered that the Gordon Korman book was not just a reading assignment, but an oral book report. "You needn't look any further," I said, "Lucas knows only too well that if he continues to be disruptive, he will be removed from your class, and what better way to get out of having to present orally without having to explain to you that he's scared to speak in front of children who laugh at him."

It occurred to me that this teacher had been with Lucas for seven months already, and yet, she knew very little about him. She should have been able to make the connection between his fear of speech and the change in his behaviour, but had not.

The school bus was another situation I had to resolve on my own. The driver had given the responsibility of monitoring the children's activities to a young girl who had a great dislike for my son. The feeling was mutual in that Lucas was then at the age when he thought all girls were ugly and stupid. Other students told me she seemed to take pleasure in reporting him for every little thing that could possibly go wrong on the way to and from school. Lucas' mouth refused to cooperate any time he would have to defend his actions to the bus driver who, understandably, could not spare the time for him to get over the blocks and the throat twisters. This led to more relaxation periods for Lucas in the principal's office. I finally put two and two together when he kept insisting I drive him to school and go pick him up.

One morning, Lucas agreed I could go with him to the bus stop to ask the other kids about the little girl who kept reporting him. Three of them confirmed what had been happening. When I reported the matter to the principal that same morning, his response was that I had to be mistaken because the young girl I was reporting to him was a high achiever and an angel. According to him, she was incapable of such conduct. Later that evening, I went to the girl's home and discussed the problem with her mother who explained that all three of her girls had their good points but there were times when their behaviour was not so perfect. I told her that the same was true about my boys.

I had also brought along some information about stuttering which certainly had a positive effect on this family as Lucas was to experience peace of mind on the bus for the rest of the year. I was surprised that this family had been so receptive to me as I discussed Lucas' problem with them, but I was relieved to know that Lucas would have one less problem to deal with. Obviously, there were still some people out there who can show sensitivity and understanding towards a child with a speech problem, and all I had to do is tell them about it.

Several other incidents occurred, far too many to discuss. What was different about our experience with this particular school and school board system was that I had finally come to the conclusion that no parent should have to work this hard at convincing educators that her child deserves the same kind of education as that offered to his fluent peers.

After approximately three months of meetings and telephone calls with school board officials, Marie Poulos eventually did meet with Lucas' teachers for the first time on April 29, 1991, and two weeks later on May 13. Unfortunately, both these meetings proved to be counterproductive and she recommended I start shopping around for another school rather than let Lucas pursue his education in an environment where it was highly unlikely that he would ever fit in.

It took me from the beginning of March to early June to get the near failing grades in oral speech adjusted on the report card. These had been attributed to Lucas by his French and his English teachers for his oral performance during the second semester. After a number of meetings with officials at the school board, it was decided that Lucas would not be given any mark at all. Given that it would have taken too much more of my time and energy to convince school and school board authorities that all I was asking for was that my child be assessed in light of his speech difficulty, I decided to simply let the matter drop.

*   *   *

At my request and subsequent to her meetings with Lucas' teachers and principal, Marie Poulos wrote the following report which she forwarded to the concerned school board authorities:

On Monday, April 29, 1991, a meeting was held to discuss the case of Lucas.

The initial phase of the meeting consisted of a review by the principal of Lucas' school history. This was followed by each teacher outlining Lucas' performance in class and any concerns regarding his speech. The French teacher commented that for the most part, Lucas' speech did not interfere significantly with his performance in class. He went on to state that Lucas tended to complete written assignments quickly and without attention to detail. Similarly, when rating his oral communication, the lower grades he assigned to Lucas were not, in his perspective, due to his speech, but to his tendency to complete oral assignments without focusing on detail.

A discussion was initiated by this therapist regarding the broader impact of Lucas' stutter not only on his speech but on his behaviour. It is possible that he may not attend to the fine details of communication both oral and written, because communication has been difficult for him. One could see a youngster communicating in any way just to get it done. In addition, a child who stutters has not had the same communication experiences as one who does not have a speech problem, so the former has a disadvantage in regard to speech practice.

The French teacher commented that Lucas has no difficulty talking or initiating speech with friends in the hallway. This therapist discussed the variability of stuttering and the fact that most people who stutter have no difficulty with familiar faces. The structured classroom environment, however, is very different than the informal speech which is carried on in a hallway.

The English teacher commented that Lucas' performance in class had been fine until the recent incidents surrounding the March oral book report presentation. She reported that, at times, he would not participate fully in discussions. She also noted that when he was required to give an oral presentation which was delayed for a few extra days, Lucas would become very anxious. She also described the types of oral communication activities she held in the classroom. These sometimes consisted of formal presentations, and more often than not, they consisted of spontaneous discussion of two to five minutes in length on a topic such as a book.

This therapist discussed stuttering hierarchies and pointed out that spontaneous discussion may be more difficult than a formal presentation. Similarly, reading is easier than other forms of speech. The principal commented that Lucas was never forced to answer a question in class, therefore, he was never under any pressure in class. This therapist pointed out that the classroom setting in general is an enormous pressure upon a youngster who cannot communicate easily or with any consistency.

In concluding, the principal said that he felt comfortable that the school had done all it could to manage Lucas' speech in the classroom. My general impression was that there is a lack of understanding of the multi-dimensional nature of stuttering and its impact on the whole person beyond his speech. The comments arising from the principal and the teachers regarding Lucas' communication, as outlined earlier in this report, indicate that further input from the speech-language pathologist is necessary to help the teachers understand and manage Lucas better in the classroom setting.

* * *

For my own piece of mind, I reported the year's events in another letter I wrote to the newly-appointed Minister of Education for the Province of Ontario, the Honourable Marion Boyd. Lucas was already registered at his new all-English school when I received her reply dated August 27, 1991. Judging from the contents of her letter below, you will note she had already been informed of our plans to move on to another system and had some excellent advice.

I am concerned by Lucas' problems and by all the difficult experiences he has encountered over the past few years. The lack of consistency in implementing remedial strategies during that time may have been detrimental to overcoming his problem.

I suggest that since your son is now registering in a new school board for the coming school year, all measures be taken from the beginning to ensure the board is fully aware of his needs, so that an appropriate program can be implemented in a consistent manner.

As you are aware, you may request an Identification, Placement and Review Committee (IPRC) meeting which will enable you to share your knowledge and experience of your son's speech problem. This will help you discuss the strategies to assist Lucas and keep you informed of his progress. I suggest you also contact the Ministry's Eastern Regional Office for more assistance.

Thank you for informing me of your concerns. I wish Lucas the best of luck in school.

* * *

CHAPTER 5

TAKING PART IN A FILM

The black cloud which had been hovering over Lucas during most of 1991 finally lifted. This time, we hit the jackpot. Thanks to some help I received from a friend, I registered Lucas in an excellent, all English school where he found peace, stability, dozens of friends and caring educators over the course of his grades 6, 7 and 8. For those of you who have lost track, my son was now on his fourth school under the jurisdiction of a third school board.

At first, I regretted enroling him in the all-English program, but finding a school which would be accepting of him was more important than pursuing a French education in systems that didn't know what to make of him. Besides, he had a French class almost every day, and could always carry on a conversation in his mother tongue with me, although when I take him up on it, he often replies: "Oh, Mother, don't you know that speaking French is so uncool!" "So sorry, no I didn't know."

I guess we are truly fortunate to live in Canada's national capital, where we have as many as five school boards. It can get confusing when one is looking for information, but as the parent of a child who stutters, I must admit I've always been grateful for the endless possibilities, not to mention that when a parent decides to move his tax dollars from one system to the next, the move is usually followed by a much better service from the education community.

Lucas' Grade 6 teacher reached out to him and offered him friendship, protection from the teasing and the support he needed to get through bad speech days. More importantly, this teacher knew how to take full advantage of a good speech day which, in turn, led to a complete turnaround in Lucas as he discovered that learning can indeed be fun. For the first time since Grade 3, he came home anxious to talk about the interesting things he was doing at his new school. What a refreshing change!

Unlike with his other schools, an Identification, Placement and Review Committee (IPRC) meeting took place in early September. Lucas' needs were formally identified and a subsequent pedagogical assessment revealed he had a lot of potential. The teacher diagnostician who conducted these tests called me herself to comment on his good nature and excellent sense of humour. Rather than labelling him as "severely learning disabled," as had been done by both of his teachers from the previous school, this specialist had taken the time to go beyond the stutter to find many of the good qualities in Lucas.

Most parents of children who stutter do not know that they can request an Identification Placement Review (IPR) case conference by which the needs of their stuttering children can be identified. Although other school systems may call it something else, whether in Canada or in the United States, this type of service is available to any parent. Not only can the needs of the child be addressed through this type of case conference, but the needs of the teacher involved in your child's education program can also be reviewed. I think the IPR process is most important in ensuring communication between the parent, the educator and the speech-language pathologist. As all three will need to work together for the benefit of a child who stutters, from the time he begins school until he feels he can handle things on his own, an IPR conference is a good place to start.

If an IPR is initiated by the parent of a child who stutters, teachers and school officials will:

- be especially sensitive to his fear of oral presentations;

- set and maintain the necessary ground rules to ensure the child's proper integration in a learning environment;

- intercept or prevent instances of ridicule and insensitivity arising from the stuttering child's manner of speech;

- acknowledge that the stuttering problem may have already been identified and adequately addressed by external specialists;

- enter into and maintain regular contact with either the school board's own speech-language pathologist or with the child's personal speech-language pathologist to ensure that the proper methods be used to help him overcome difficult speech-related situations at school;

- assess the child's oral performance in light of his speech difficulty;

- give the child the options to either submit an oral assignment on audio cassette, or to present in front of his teacher only, or in front of a small group of students who do not find stuttering amusing;

- help the child who stutters make gradual steps towards an oral presentation in front of the entire class; and

- call on him early in class to avoid undue stress as he anticipates his turn to speak.

* * *

Also in September, 1990, Lucas received a special telephone call from his friend Dave Taylor. Dave was in town along with the rest of his teammates for their annual training camp event held at the Bob Guertin arena in Hull, Quebec, just across the Ottawa River from our home town. He was inviting us to come and join him in the press box to watch the L.A. Kings at practice. What an evening this was for all of us, especially for my husband Paul and my eldest son Jonathan, the true hockey fanatics in our family and who had not met Dave in Anaheim, California.

I remember how disappointed Jonathan was because I couldn't afford to take both of them with me to the National Stuttering Project (NSP) conference on stuttering the year before. Jonathan had been so envious that when Lucas came home with Dave's hockey stick, he complained it wasn't really fair for his younger brother to get all the goods just because of his stuttering!

Well, finally I was able to make things right again with Jonathan. Dave asked them both to join him in the press box, giving them each their own special autographed L.A. Kings ball cap. Jonathan who is normally shy with new people, but who doesn't stutter, chatted incessantly with Dave when he joined us in the stands.

As if that wasn't enough excitement for the boys, Dave took them to meet the owner of the Kings at the time, Bruce McNall, and Larry Robinson who also gave them his autograph. Jonathan and Lucas couldn't believe their good fortune and the whole evening had been a great boost to their egos. Just as I suspected, there were no problems getting the boys off to school the next morning. I can attest to the fact that they got there at least some twenty minutes before everyone else. Both wanted to make sure they would have enough time to do a bit of bragging, and in Lucas' case especially, why not!

In early October, I had to undergo major surgery. I was recuperating in hospital when I noticed my husband Paul was unusually quiet during one of his visits. I immediately thought something must have happened to one of the boys, but it had nothing to do with them. The disturbing news I was about to hear left me feeling numb all over; Marie Poulos, Lucas' personal speech-language pathologist, had died tragically in an automobile crash, the day before on October 6, 1991.

Arrangements were made so I could be released from hospital as soon as possible because Paul and I both felt it best that I be the one to tell Lucas. The news of Marie's death was being broadcast on radio and television, and we worried that Lucas would find out before I had a chance to talk to him. I made it home on October 8, and that same morning I received a call from the principal informing me that school officials were keeping a close eye on my son to make sure he didn't go anywhere in the school where he could hear or see a news broadcast about Marie's accident.

Lucas was surprised to find me home in bed when he arrived from his day at school. There was no easy way to tell him so I tried to do it as quickly as possible so it wouldn't hurt as much. "It's OK to cry," I said.

Born in Belleville, Ontario, Marie graduated from Belleville Collegiate and went on to receive a Masters degree in speech pathology at the University of Toronto. Throughout the 1980's and up until her death, she ran a successful stuttering therapy program at the Rehabilitation Centre in Ottawa, Ontario, which helped hundreds of persons who stutter from all across Canada. The program which Marie set up has been recognized as a model of its kind because of its success in dealing with the problem of relapse after the initial intensive treatment. Follow-up sessions, refresher courses, and a self-help group have been major factors in the continued success of her clients a decade later. Many have gone on to be excellent communicators in a number of walks of life demanding precision speaking skills.

(The above was excerpted from a press release prepared by Michael Petrunik, Ph.D., Faculty of Social Sciences, University of Ottawa. Michael had been a patient and a friend of Marie's.)

I knew that in Lucas' heart, no one would ever be able to take her place. At times, when I see him struggle to get a word out, I think of Marie and how I miss her. Not only had she untangled his tongue, but she had given him a new lease on life.

*   *   *

November was a particularly special time, because a Toronto film crew travelled to Ottawa to shoot Lucas' segment for *Speaking of Courage*, a documentary on stuttering which was dedicated to the memory of Marie Poulos. She would have been proud of the significant contributions made to this special film project by some of her patients.

The school's administration staff and Lucas' teacher were very receptive to the camera crew, and the Grade 6 students were both proud and delighted to take part in what turned out to be a good learning experience for all.

*   *   *

I wrote the following story as my way of saying thanks to the Toronto film crew.

Lights, Camera and . . . Action! . . . Our moment in the spotlight came to an end this week. Now I know that making movies isn't as glamorous as one would expect. As a matter-of-fact, it was downright stressful at times. The crew returned to Toronto with some 38 hours of film footage to be edited for a one-hour program. We will have to wait until next fall to see the end product.

Lucas was filmed at school, there was a teacher and principal interview, a dinner scene filmed at the house, a bus scene (for which a city bus was chartered) and other interviews at home with both my boys, Lucas and Jonathan, and then with my husband Paul and I. Thanks to Jonathan's strong organizational skills, several of the boys' friends were recruited to be filmed in a street hockey game. Lucas' older brother really gave it his best shot, assigning positions based on proven skill and ability and he also prepared a diagram indicating the names of his players.

The scene was shot at a nearby park and was pretty special in itself. Normally, when children gather in front of our house to play, all you can hear are screams of excitement, and of course, there's always the occasional fight. For the film though, all the producer got was silence. Members of the crew had to assume the role of screaming coaches to snap them out of it.

The bus scene turned out to be an interesting event as well. Our bus service had been cut off for the past few months, and here was a city bus right on the street to pick up Lucas at the door. Not only that, the bus was in showroom condition: I had never seen such a good-looking machine! I had to run around at the last minute to find extras for the bus ride to school that morning. Six of our neighbours were more than happy to oblige.

Everyone looked just smashing, including the bus driver in his impeccable uniform. The bus went up and down the street several times with the cameraman hanging out the window of the crew's van which travelled alongside it to get a special shot of Lucas through the bus window. He was told to appear deep in thought. What an actor! Hollywood here we come!

Inviting a camera crew into your home can cause quite a stir. Every time they marched in with their equipment, I wondered how would I ever put everything back in place. They would literally tear a room apart and rearrange all the furniture to set up. They would grab stuff from the other rooms to create just the right atmosphere in one place, and start all over again in another room.

I thought filming a dinner scene would be easy, but trying to serve, think, talk and look in the right direction all at the same time was a very difficult thing to do. By the time this particular scene came about, my boys had already been exposed to the camera and certainly did much better than I, except I found it strange to hear Jonathan reply, "Yes, Maam," when I asked him if he had a good day at school.

I guess he was trying to be extra polite. Unusual, but certainly polite. Had we accidentally stumbled onto something great here . . . ? I wondered if I could convince the crew to keep the camera rolling in this house until Jonathan turned, uum . . . let's say 21? Yes, that would be very helpful in getting me through the terrible teen years.

There was a television monitor set up in the living room to observe what was going on in the kitchen. At one point, someone yelled out for me to STOP EATING! I should have been warned to eat just little bits at a time because if they had to reshoot, all the plates on the table had to be refilled to the exact amount of food left on them when the filming stopped. When it was finally over, I was stuffed. There was no point in trying to explain I usually have a small appetite, no one would have believed me. One of the crew members later mentioned that the dinner scene in *Moonstruck* took two weeks to shoot. I thought it kind of him to provide me with that little titbit of movie information.

My interview had been scheduled for the following day. I must have done alright, although I was not prepared for some of the questions which were put to me. The crew was friendly, and they did a lot of kidding around, but once the camera started to roll, they meant business. I started to sweat under those lights after a while. It may be hard for some to believe (especially those who know me well), but I did remain calm for most of the two-hour interview.

The issues surrounding some of the problems Lucas experienced at school were difficult to discuss on film. A box of Kleenex came in handy at one point . . . and not just for me! A quick exit to the crisp air outside did wonders to help me regain my composure. It's a good thing I'm not involved in any of the editing because once I'd get through cutting, there wouldn't be much film left to work with.

The crew wrapped things up with a final interview in the living room with Paul and me. Although he does not particularly enjoy taking part in any form of public speaking activity, my husband did great. I found it more enjoyable to do an interview with him beside me. It's easier when there are two people to think of just the right answer.

Special thanks to Vladimir Bondarenko, Producer, David Lancaster, Manager, Jim Borecki, Cameraman, Brian Kaulback, Assistant, and Peter Sawade, Soundman. *Speaking of Courage* will be instrumental in bringing about some much needed changes in our Canadian education system for all the beautiful children who live with a stutter.

*   *   *

Speaking of Courage was presented for the first time on television on March 3, 1993. TVOntario aired it a second time in July of that same year. Since then, the documentary has won the Silver Apple Award at the National Educational Film and Video Festival in California, and it was nominated for a Golden Sheaf Award at the Yorkton Festival in Saskatchewan (Canada). More recently, Vladimir Bondarenko's work as the film's Producer and Director also earned him a nomination for Best Director at the Gemini Awards held in Toronto on March 3, 1994. These awards are Canada's equivalent to the Emmy Awards in the U.S.

The one-hour film explores the depth to which stuttering pervades every moment in the lives of people who stutter, and leaves the audience with a deeper understanding and appreciation of its nature and often devastating impact. This video is hosted and narrated by acclaimed Canadian actress Sheila McCarthy, whose father stuttered all his life.

[For information on how to obtain a copy of the video, see the Reference Guide.]

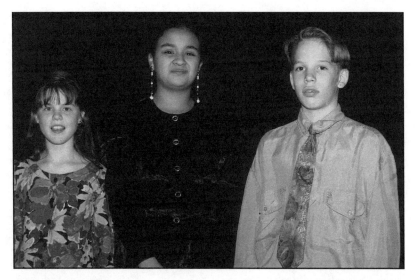

The children of *Speaking of Courage,* Alyssa Young of Clarksburg, Carolina Ayala of Toronto, Ontario, and Lucas (not so comfortable in the company of girls!).

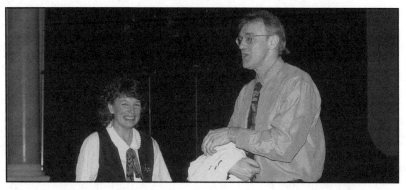

Mom is presented with her *Speaking of Courage* T-shirt at the Ottawa Film Premiere held at the Chateau Laurier Hotel.

The second story I wrote about the film was published in the April 1992 edition of a Toronto-based magazine called *Abilities*. This article talks about a very special group of friends who made significant contributions to the making of the film *Speaking of Courage.*

The Ontario Barber Shop Singers Harmonize for Speech . . . One percent of the adult population and four percent of the children of the Western world stutter. Despite its widespread recognition, much ignorance and many myths remain a part of the public misunderstanding of this communication disorder.

Unfortunately for children who stutter, attending school often becomes an experience of ridicule, fear, teacher and peer insensitivity, anger, frustration and helplessness. However, as the general public, and more importantly, educators, doctors and politicians learn more about stuttering, dysfluency in children will begin to receive the empathy and understanding it deserves.

Three years ago, my son Lucas and I were given a special opportunity to take part in a film called *Speaking of Courage*. When we were first contacted by the Toronto film producer, Vladimir Bondarenko, he explained he was working on a human-interest documentary about people who stutter. This project was sponsored in part by the *Harmonize for Speech Fund* of the *Ontario Barber Shop Singers*.

The film was a first attempt in Canada to focus on stuttering in children and to present dysfluency to the general public who would view the project. By participating, we realized we could also help others who live with this difficulty.

At first, I was hesitant about going public with our personal situation, but when I was told of other families willing to share their experience, I was confident this project would work. After years of trying to make people understand this neurologically-based disorder, it was a nice feeling knowing we were not alone. I knew this film project was the best possible means of creating greater awareness of the problems and frustrations people who stutter encounter in everyday living.

Although difficult at times, our opportunity to improve the quality of life of dysfluent children remains an experience we will treasure for a long time to come. In spite of his battle with his tongue, Lucas enjoyed working with the crew and his embarrassment at making himself understood gradually disappeared.

In early January, 1992, when the filming had been completed, the parents of three of the children featured in the film were given the chance to express their gratitude to the barbershoppers for their generous contributions to the project. The families travelled to Orillia, Ontario, where the sponsors held their annual conference. During a special ceremony which took place on Saturday, January, 11, Paul and Daphne Young mentioned how grateful they were for the barbershoppers' donation towards their daughter Alyssa's speech therapy. They added it had given their family a sense of dignity and they were encouraged just knowing that others felt the needs of their child were worth fighting for.

The parents of 13-year-old Carolina Ayala delivered their thank you speeches in Spanish. Although no one else in the auditorium spoke the language, what they were saying was unmistakably clear to us all.

The determination displayed by Carolina as she translated her parents' words, and added a few of her own, was a truly emotional experience. As I stood by her mother, I couldn't help feeling the mixture of pride and anguish we mothers experience when we watch our children trying to express themselves. Normally, I am just as scared as Lucas whenever he must speak in front of strangers who may not know how to react to his disability, but it was obvious I had nothing to fear in this room filled with nearly 300 barber shop singers. As with the other children, Lucas' short speech was well-received.

Following the presentation of *Speaking of Courage* on television, I received many letters from individuals who were impressed and deeply moved by the film. I would like to share two of these letters with you.

The first was written by David Radcliffe, Associate Dean, Faculty of Education, The University of Western Ontario.

As you heard on the phone, my stutter today is most of the time almost undetectable. Both I and my elder brother stutter. His form of stuttering is a moderately severe speech hesitancy, but mine was a total shut-down. One might say his brakes are half on, and grabbing, whereas mine were totally locked. My parents were told that his problem was less severe – at least he could get something out – but mine was the more difficult to deal with.

In my school years, I was sent to see a distinguished British speech therapist, Dr. Lionel Logue. Logue was the therapist for George VI, and I remember him saying, "Did you hear my King last week?" after the King had given a public speech, or radio address. Always, with great pride, "my King." I can imagine him listening to a royal address like a back-seat driver, willing "his King," over the difficult bits. Logue saw the problem as mechanical, and prescribed a series of syllabic exercises, with tricks for getting the words out. He was a wonderful and caring person, but it did not really help me.

When I was an undergraduate student at Cambridge University, I went to see a therapist associated with Addenbrookes Hospital. Her approach was quite different. She began by assuring me that there was absolutely nothing mechanically wrong; mouth, throat, tongue, larynx, etc. were all in proper working order. I think that this is sometimes a worry for young children who stutter. Then basically, she prescribed simple breathing exercises and relaxation techniques. It worked for me. The key was the relaxation for its own sake. I can let my body go, flop out, so completely that it sometimes takes a moment or two to get it moving again.

However, my stutter still comes back when I am tired or physically run down. And there are some things I cannot do with ease. I cannot readily join in a lively conversation; I can't butt in. I am often the quiet one in any academic seminar or discussion, forced to keep my thoughts and insights to myself, which is not a good professional trait. I can't tell a good joke (unless I am putting on a dialect) because that punch line is lying in wait to trip me up.

I am sometimes in difficulties on the telephone, particularly when the person at the other end seems to be dominating the conversation. Unless they know me, because they cannot see that I am in difficulties, they get impatient. "Hello, hello, – pause – Are you still there? – must have rung off!" and down goes the phone. I have to call back, and if I am now relaxed enough, I apologize for the problem and blame the telephone company for some sort of mechanical failure!

One thing I think is very useful, is a sense of humour. As I said, both my brother and I stutter, and we can recognise other people who stutter. There are many forms, some of which fluent people might not notice or perceive as stuttering. Dr. Rob Buckman (host of the TVOntario program called *Vital Signs* during which *Speaking of Courage* was presented) will have known Magnus Pyke, who had a wonderful TV series on popular science some years ago, also carried by TVO. Pyke's stutter was manifested mainly in extravagant gesticulation.

I remember that my brother and I used to imitate other people who stutter in the privacy of our shared bedroom, and it was often hilarious. "Have you heard this kind?" or "Have you seen people who go like this?" It sounds cruel and heartless, except when you remember that we both stuttered ourselves, and that it was a way of dealing with our pain and embarrassment.

It is a curious fact that many people who stutter can step outside themselves and be quite clever mimics. I noticed this in the TVO film, when that very courageous young girl was quoting and imitating her parents and her teacher in her prepared speech. I think that people who stutter become quite observant, both of others and of themselves, and this can be turned to good advantage. My brother has a wonderful command of British regional dialects and accents, and is a great raconteur.

So more power to you in what you are doing and to your son.

The second letter was from Margo of Sarnia, Ontario.

> My letter is to the children featured in the film *Speaking of Courage*.
> My name is Margo and I am 39 years old. I stuttered when I was
> younger and over the years, I overcame this prison to which I am
> able to relate so very much with all of you.
>   Watching that film moved me to many tears, and I once again
> felt as if I was a child back in school experiencing the frustration,
> hurt and pain that only we can understand.
>   I want to encourage each of you to continue with your speech
> therapy sessions, keep practising, and you will conquer this prob-
> lem. I will be thinking of you.

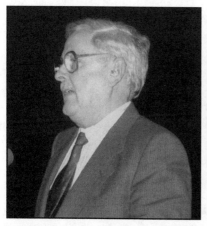

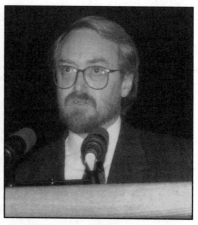

Jock Carlise, author of *Tangled Tongue* and
who is also featured in *Speaking of Courage*.

David Lancaster, Manager, gives a bit of
history about the film at the Ottawa Premiere.

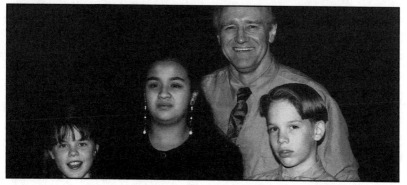

Vladimir Bondarenko, producer of *Speaking of Courage*, with the children.

CHAPTER 6

STUTTERING AND THE TEENAGE YEARS

On his last day of school in June 1991, the first thing Lucas said to me when he got home was that there would be no need for him to go and meet his Grade 7 teachers in August. Grade 6 had been a great experience; he got good marks and he felt confident enough to go to his first day of school next September without having to worry about how new people would react to his stutter. How I looked forward to the anxiety-free summer! However, I suspected he would probably feel differently come mid-August.

When he started asking a lot of questions about how he would cope on his first day of Junior High, it was obvious that he was becoming apprehensive. He knew he would be rotating from class to class, and it had finally dawned on him that there would be at least eight new teachers to meet during his first week of school. As he kept reminding me how difficult it was going to be for him, and how he wished he could go back to having just one teacher again, I called the principal and made an appointment for Lucas to meet his home room teacher.

The child in him was in a state of panic at home, but the teen who accompanied me to this meeting presented a very different facade to the new principal and homeroom teacher. In fact, he made his mother look like she had dragged him there against his will. On our way back to the car in the school's parking lot, my son reverted to his old self again, so I asked, "What was that all about in there?" "Nothing," he replied. "Nothing, simply won't do," I said, "because I've never seen you act like this before, so out with it." He didn't have to say anything, the look he gave me was all too familiar to me.

A couple of years ago, I had gone through the same thing with Jonathan who began to feel embarrassed about being seen just about anywhere with his mother. I was thinking how much easier it will be to communicate with my boys once they reach adulthood when Lucas managed to say "It just felt strange going to meet my teacher with you there." Grateful there wasn't anything else to it, I told him he was forgiven and that I understood completely. I lied, however; this was another one of those times when his feelings took priority over mine.

As with every other child who begins Junior High, switching from the one-room setting to rotating from class to class, took some time to get used to. By Christmas, Lucas seemed to have settled down nicely. He was involved in a short-lived relationship with his first girlfriend which led to several interesting chats with Mom.

I was glad my warnings against a major commitment at his young age had some effect in that he continues to be involved in sports and other activities which are also essential to his growing up. As he loves to dance, he's still very popular with the girls, but he is not letting it interfere with anything else he would rather do. I realize things may change over time. Hopefully, I will be ready for those changes when they occur.

Like many other boys their age, mine have also been involved in minor incidences of mischief. I suppose they wouldn't be normal if they hadn't. While Jonathan knew which buttons to push to drive any teacher mad, there were times when Lucas was also found guilty of similar misconduct. I recall a particular situation which turned out to be another learning experience for both Lucas and me.

One evening, I received a telephone call from his science teacher who informed me that my son had not reported to the lab for some unfinished business. The teacher wanted him to clean up the liquid detergent which had been spilled on the classroom floor. As the other parties involved had decided to skip detention, Lucas also made a quick exit after class. Being left alone to clean up the mess didn't exactly seem fair to him. His teacher asked that I bring him to the school's administration office the next morning.

Letter of apology in hand, Lucas looked pretty sheepish standing face to face, or should I say face to belt buckle, with his teacher who was still annoyed with him. I couldn't blame the teacher for being angry, after all, he's the one who ended up having to clean up the mess himself before he went home. I meant to suggest we move to a more private location instead of standing in the middle of heavy student and teacher traffic in the school's main office, but I kept quiet thinking another detention would be assigned and this whole scene would be over in a matter of minutes.

Lucas kept his eyes to the floor the whole time his teacher questioned him about his disappearing act the night before. His loud tone was heard by several around us. I knew my son's speech would not cooperate in this type of circumstance, and I was not surprised to see him standing there with his mouth open for what seemed to be an eternity. I felt sorry for Lucas, who never did get to explain why he had skipped detention, however, I was most disturbed by the look of disgust displayed by the teacher. He seemed upset with the child for not being able to respond to him.

Any other time, I would have interrupted and explained that it would be highly unlikely that my son would be able to get a syllable out, never mind a complete word, if the teacher continued to look at him so strangely. Lucas wasn't even looking at him, so I didn't bother. The week before, I had been angered when a salesman at an electronics store gave my son and his friend Norm the exact same look when they were out doing speech transfer activities at a local shopping mall. I had said nothing then either. Could it be that I was starting to mellow? Not quite.

Having served his detention, Lucas was late getting home that evening. It was a quiet supper. Things are always quiet when he's mad. I thought I'd give him a chance to come around on his own before I asked how his day had gone, and it was practically his bedtime before I got around to asking. I was secretly hoping he would still be mad because his speech is always fluent is such circumstances, and we could get to the root of the problem more quickly.

My first question was: "Is there a reason why you don't seem to like this teacher as much as the others?" Bingo! "I can't stand him," Lucas screamed, "every time he asks me to talk in class, he looks at me as if I'm retarded or something!"

Trying to minimize the importance of those incidents, I said: "Is that all?" Bad move. This triggered an even louder screaming episode before I could get him to calm down. Finally, I told him I had observed the strange looks from his teacher, and agreed he was justified in being angry with him, but spilling liquids in this teacher's class would only bring him further away from resolving the situation in a satisfactory manner. It was getting late, so I told him to get some sleep while I thought of some way to fix this problem. He didn't have to go back to this teacher's class for a couple of days, so we had time to come up with an idea.

Over the weekend, I came up with the perfect plan to help him. As it turned out, extra bonus marks could be obtained in this teacher's class if students clipped out newspaper articles related to the subject matter taught, summarized them in their own words and presented them in a neat format. I told my son I could easily go to the school and discuss the situation with his teacher, and if that didn't work, I could take it up with the principal. But he and I both knew this could lead to other problems. I warned that the teacher might not appreciate being told he makes faces and could, in turn, make Lucas' life miserable for the rest of the year.

And besides, I felt strongly that the teacher wasn't even aware of what he was doing and its effect on Lucas.

A couple of weeks before all this happened, I had been interviewed by Paul Taylor, a medical reporter from Toronto. Following this telephone interview, Mr. Taylor wrote an excellent article on stuttering which appeared in *The Globe and Mail.* It took some doing to convince Lucas that this article was indeed related and, finally, he agreed to summarize it in such a way as to resolve his latest problem without having to confront his teacher. With a few helpful hints from Mom, Lucas dropped off the following paper in his teacher's mail slot first thing Monday morning:

> This article is about me because it talks about stuttering. Stuttering is like a short circuit in the brain. In the article, Dr. Kroll says it's a *coordination deficit*, but I still say it's like a short circuit in the brain.
>
> At first, scientists thought kids who stuttered did it because they had bad parents, like Professor Johnson said in the 1950's. Now we know better.
>
> Dr. Webster who says something in this article too, has done a lot of research on stuttering. He is a scientist who used to live in Ottawa. Now he lives in St. Catharines, Ontario. He knows all about the Precision Fluency Shaping Program (PFSP) and what it can do for people who stutter. The PFSP is the program I took a couple of years ago to learn how to control my speech. There is no cure for stuttering, so doing speech targets is the best thing anyone who stutters can do.
>
> All the doctors and professors in this article are the best specialists in our whole country. They know the most about stuttering. A lot of work needs to be done because people still don't know what to do when they meet someone who stutters. Maybe some day people will stop laughing or making faces at stuttering, and maybe people won't find stuttering so strange when they know more about it.

Lucas never did bring home this assignment to show me his bonus mark, but there were no more incidents of strange faces.

During a meeting I had with Allan Peterkin, M.D. from the University of Ottawa's Health Services, I mentioned this particular story and how we had managed to resolve the problem. The psychiatrist and published author of children's books was looking for some information about a child who stutters for a story he was working on at the time. He commented on my innovative plan which showed Lucas he had a variety

of other means at his disposal to resolve unfortunate situations surrounding his speech.

*   *   *

"Ages thirteen to eighteen are cited as the most difficult times for speech
therapy because teenagers are more self-conscious about themselves.
Dating, skin problems, and impressing the opposite sex become more
important to them than confronting stuttering. University of Western
Ontario Professor William Yovetich says this is when kids try to hide
stuttering the most and the stage at which most students drop out of
speech therapy."[1]

For the teenager who stutters, denial of his handicap may also bring
about some significant changes in his behaviour. Lucas was no exception. I wrote this next story shortly after he made the decision not to go
back to speech class.

Thinking Things Through . . . Lucas has been an unwilling participant in
speech therapy for some time now. He lost all interest after the accidental death of his personal speech-language pathologist, Marie, who, for
over two years had had a tremendous impact on his life. I continued to
help him with his speech exercises at home, but it was getting more and
more difficult to get him to cooperate. Needless to say, he always had
something better to do.

More than a full year had gone by before a new speech-language
pathologist was hired to take over Marie's position at the Rehabilitation
Centre here in Ottawa, Ontario. Lucas was scheduled to meet with
Carol Bock for an initial session, and for some strange reason, he was
not happy to go. I couldn't figure out if his behaviour was just another
one of those terrible teen reactions, or if he feared finding out how much
work he had ahead of him to get his speech skills back to where they were
several months ago. He was asked to come for a second visit and, this
time, he was mad at me for taking him.

Seeing how reluctant he was, Carol suggested a contract be drawn
up between the three of us to make sure the home exercises got done.
All three of us agreed that if he did not hold up to his end of the bargain,
the contract could be torn up. As bribing him with a chocolate bar, a
variety of other treats or a special outing no longer worked with my
13-year old, I went through several weeks of trying to reason with him.

Nothing seemed to work, so I asked him to write a letter to Carol inform- ing her that he would not be going to speech therapy any more. No more hard work, no more techniques, no more nothing.

We discussed his decision at length. I told him that even though I did not agree with it, I would respect his wishes to discontinue his ther- apy. I hurt inside when I hear him grunt, but I said nothing. Grunting happens to be his latest thing. Not only does he grunt to clear the blocks, he has also developed several new voices to ensure a smoother flow of speech.

He has obviously discovered that if he uses a voice other than his own, he can achieve some level of fluency. He is not very successful at it, but he thinks that he is, and I suppose that's all that matters. What is especially bizarre with this new voice trick of his is that there are times when I could swear I am listening to a cartoon on television. Perhaps I should keep a record of Lucas' new experiments which seem to surface on a weekly basis.

I spoke to his new speech-language pathologist just the other day. Carol seemed as disappointed as I, but she told me what Lucas was doing right now is typical of teenagers who stutter. My main concern was the impact that my son's new self-imposed fluency tactics could have on his speech, and would they cause irreparable damage. Marie had once told me that secondary or accessory behaviours which Lucas often used to delay his stuttering could be difficult to undo, but Carol assured me that they wouldn't. She planned to contact Lucas in a few more days to let him know she will be there for him should he decide to go back to ther- apy.

It's been a difficult week. Now that we've all had a chance to think things through, it would appear (at least for the time being) that leaving therapy was the route to take.

* * *

My article was published in the NSP's *Letting Go* Newsletter. Two weeks later, I received some correspondence from Carl Dell Jr., Ph.D., author of *Treating the School-Aged Stutterer, a Guide for Clinicians,* and Assistant Professor in speech pathology and audiology at Eastern Illinois Univer- sity.

Dr. Dell and I had met briefly at the June 1990 conference on stut- tering in Anaheim, California. I was grateful for his words of encouragement which can also be appreciated by all parents of teenagers who stutter.

I was sure moved by your caring and sensitive article regarding your son, Lucas. I think parents suffer from stuttering much more than the children. It's not unlike watching your children participate in athletics. My wife Margaret and I get much more nervous watching our son, Adam, than I ever experienced as a player. We feel so helpless and we want everything to go just right for our children, however, it's a good thing everything doesn't go right for our kids because if it did, they wouldn't learn anything. Failure and some suffering are necessary for growth, and without it, we couldn't reach our full potential. The prettiest flower is often found in the rocky places rather than in the well-manicured garden.

Lucas is struggling. Those teenage years are tough enough without stuttering to complicate things. Yes, he's struggling and he knows all these little tricks he is using are hard on his feelings of self worth. He knows he should have the courage to speak up and not resort to tricks, but stuttering is so embarrassing, and it's hard to be the warrior all the time.

How well I remember those teenage years. Trying by all manner of trickery to hide my stuttering. Hating speech therapy because it reminded me I was different. My great fear was that the other kids would find out I was in therapy. And then my dirty little secret would be out in the open. People who stutter are so unrealistic in one sense. We have this feeling that we can hide stuttering when in reality, everyone knows we stutter. We go to such great lengths to pretend we're fluent, when people already know the truth.

I was just becoming a good athlete by the time I was at Lucas' age. I remember being able to prove myself on the ball field, and how great that made me feel. I know Lucas is interested in sports; I hope he works hard enough to become good at something. I know it really helped me combat all the negatives I felt about stuttering.

I realized that hard work led to improved skills in sport, but in contrast, hard work on my speech didn't lead as dramatically to improvement. No matter how much I tried, I couldn't will myself or practice enough to stop stuttering. Stuttering seemed to have a life of its own, and I couldn't overcome it in spite of tireless effort. It caused me a lot of frustration. I couldn't understand how I could try so hard and still fail. It didn't seem to happen that way in sports. Yes, I lost at times or played poorly, but practice did help me improve. I never could get that same feeling with stuttering.

I usually encourage parents of youngsters to bring them to therapy despite their resistance. Usually, when these kids see that speech-language pathologists are non-threatening and non-judgemental, they soon come to like our visits together. I still tell parents to bring them in, but will let the child make his own decision after a few sessions. It we can't convince him we have something that will benefit him, then we are probably wasting time forcing him to be in therapy.

As I've written and talked about so often before, stuttering is so frustrating. I can be fluent when alone, or at times when I'm with others. But I can't count on it. And this sometimes fluency makes me feel like such a failure when I do stutter. Why can't I be fluent all the time? To some extent, the asthmatic says the same thing, "Why can't I always breathe easily?" The difference is that people who stutter and their families feel that continual fluency is possible with more effort or more confidence.

This is, of course, the great misconception of stuttering. However, it is true that continually practising a technique may diminish the stuttering, but usually will not totally extinguish it. All of us would then reason that improvement is worth the price of continual vigilance. But for people who stutter and for young children in particular, this improvement in speech may not be worth the price. Speech is meant to be spontaneous and free, not guarded and regulated.

Kids resent all this attention over their speech. It's similar to asking adults to change their breathing from the normal 12 breaths per minute to 10 for example. You would keep up this need to continually monitor respiration for a period of time, but eventually, you would grow weary of the constant attention to something that we all do spontaneously. Talking is fun, but people who stutter in therapy are forced to undergo hard labour if they are to successfully control their stuttering. The whole idea of control, is indeed completely foreign to the act of speech, and yet we ask our children to control and monitor an activity which doesn't easily lend itself to being controlled.

I also remember that stuttering wasn't then, nor is it now the focus of my life. It is one branch of the tree that is Carl Dell. It is no more than that. I refuse to let stuttering interfere with what I want to do with my life. The same was true when I was 13. Stuttering was really a minor nuisance. Like the fat girl or the short boy, it was something I wished was not there, but like other kids, I could learn to cope and be accepted in spite of my flaws.

I understand your pain. Know that you are not alone. You and Lucas are part of our family, and if we can be of any service, please don't hesitate to call or write.

*   *   *

This was one letter I wanted to share with Lucas who, after reading it, said: "I like this guy, he's on my side!"

Note

1. Sutter, Paul J. 1994. *In a Manner of Speaking: Strategies for Stutterers.* Today's Parent. November 1994 Edition. Pages 102-103 and 104.

CHAPTER 7

TIPS FOR THE PARENT AND THE TEACHER

Parents of children who stutter realize teachers have a difficult job to do. They are equally aware of the time pressures teachers face on a daily basis, and more importantly, parents know how trying it is for their stuttering children to cope in a learning environment where the major focus remains on effective communication.

Children who stutter can be identified by their typical behavioral patterns. For example, when they are asked to perform orally in front of a group or when asked a question in class, they will most likely give teachers a short reply, like a *YES* or a *NO*, or even *I DON'T KNOW*, anything to get the teacher to move on to the next student as quickly as possible. In doing so, they can avoid further exposure as students who cannot speak as well as the others.

As their minds appear to be programmed to give out short replies, some of these children also have a tendency to do the same when it comes to producing their written assignments. What better motivation to keep sentences short than the fear of being asked to read them aloud in class?

Another interesting factor to be considered is that children who stutter may demonstrate poor organizational skills; if school represents a stressful environment for them, they will probably do all that they can to tune themselves out. One can understand how easy it is for a teacher to identify this *Tuning Out Syndrome* as a total lack of interest on the part of his/her student. Finally, there are several other common denominators to be found in dysfluent children, all of which can be discussed with the child's parent and/or personal speech-language pathologist.

For the child who stutters, the road to fluency represents a lot of hard work. Dysfluent kids know what is involved in achieving success with the use of just one particular speech target. Techniques to control a stutter take considerable effort and skill which should not go unnoticed. While most of us take speech for granted, children who stutter will tell you that fluency is *easier done than said*.

Many educators have asked me what are the targets to look for in the speech of a child who has undergone therapy. Listed below are seven speech targets normally used by graduates of intensive treatment programs. The name of each target may vary slightly from one treatment program to the next, but can still be easily identified by the patient. The following definitions were given to me in the form of a hand-out at one of Lucas' refresher courses.

Before I list the techniques, it is important to note that those used by my son do not necessarily apply to ALL children. Lucas' skills were learned in a structured environment, and it took a long time before his therapist and I could expect that he would *transfer* his acquired fluency skills to the classroom. It would be best for teachers to maintain contact with the speech-language pathologist and the parent to be aware of the child's progress in therapy and of the techniques which are most helpful to him.

Although fluency-shaping techniques are the ones most often used in therapy, there are others which are preferred for certain children, depending on the various types and severity of stuttering, of course.

Once the fluency techniques have been identified, their use should be encouraged by teachers to help the student make a smoother transition from the clinical setting to the classroom.

1. The **STRETCHED SYLLABLE** consists of stretching speech sounds beyond their normal value. The application of the stretched syllable speech target ensures that movements occur slowly enough to notice, and to alter them in a deliberate manner if need be. It also provides a vehicle into which new types of speech movements can be transferred. It can be achieved by placing the articulators in position for the first sound of the syllable; that position is held for two seconds with a gradual shift of the muscles enabling the production of the remainder of the syllable.

2. The **FULL BREATH** speech target will help rectify the following possible errors in breathing such as speaking with an inadequate air supply, exhaling before speaking, quick, shallow breaths, saying too much on one breath or inhaling with shoulders or upper chest. It is achieved by taking a slow, comfortable inhalation using the diaphragm. The patient/student will then begin exhaling and speaking at the same time, without any hesitation between the inhalation and the exhalation. You will note a gradual relaxation of the diaphragm as the child speaks. Once complete relaxation of the diaphragm is achieved, the child knows to stop talking, take a short pause and begin another breath.

3. The **GENTLE ONSET** is the **most important target** of the program. It involves initiating speech with low amplitude vibrations of the vocal folds followed by smoothly increasing the strength of those vibrations. It is achieved by taking a slow, comfortable inhalation with a gradual increase in the strength of the vibrations until the normal loudness level is reached. You will note a slight reduction in the strength of the vibrations at the end of a syllable.

4. **SLOW CHANGE** is the slow movement of muscles from one articulatory position to another. The method is achieved by stretching the first sound for its entire duration as the strength of the vocal fold vibrations is increased. Before the patient reaches his strongest vibrations (normal loudness), he will move his articulators slowly and smoothly to the sound that follows.

5. **REDUCED AIR PRESSURE** is the speech target which will result in a reduction of the air flow passing through the vocal tract. It will ensure that the onset of the following sound is gradual and gentle.

6. The **REDUCED ARTICULATORY PRESSURE** is achieved by reducing the tension and the pressure in the lips and tongue to a minimum. Conversely, increased articulatory pressure will prevent voicing from beginning gently.

7. The **AMPLITUDE CONTOUR TARGET** will ensure correct initiation of syllables which follow the first and will help in the maintenance of voicing. The method is achieved by reducing the loudness/strength of the vocal fold vibrations at the end of each syllable and by beginning the following syllable gently. The patient is taught not to pause between syllables, except to take a breath as necessary.

Speech therapy sounds complicated, doesn't it? It is. Not only does the person who stutters have to master the use of the individual speech targets or various combinations of one or two of these techniques, but they must also learn the Class Sounds to which each target is applicable.

*   *   *

As the parent of a child who stutters, you can expect that teachers will want to ask you what they can do to help. When faced with such a request, parents should take advantage of the situation as this will give them an excellent opportunity to open the lines of communication between parent, teacher and speech-language pathologist. If all three work together to help the student feel more open and comfortable about his stuttering, many unfortunate incidents can be diminished or avoided altogether.

The following has been excerpted from a publication produced by the Curriculum Resource Department of the Metropolitan Separate School Board, Toronto, Ontario. *The Student who Stutters: Some questions and answers* was prepared by Julie Mazzuca-Peter, speech-language pathologist.

When the classroom teacher is confronted with a student who stutters, s/he may not know how to react. Sometimes, in an honest effort to help, teachers are often perplexed because a stuttering child becomes more shy, less talkative and responsive to their efforts. Speech interruptions may become more frequent and pronounced.

Would it be best to supply words as soon as any stuttering commences? Should the student be reassured that it doesn't matter that s/he has trouble when reciting? Should s/he be excused from oral presentations and oral responses, and be allowed to do extra written assignments? Or is it best to ignore the stuttering altogether and pretend it doesn't exist?

Here are some answers to the more commonly asked questions teachers have:

What should I do when a student in my class stutters?

Listen to what s/he says, not how s/he says it. Let the student take all the time s/he needs to make a point. Don't ask him/her to *slow down* or *relax* – you will only draw attention away from the topic to the speech difficulty.

Should I excuse the student from oral presentation of projects or reports?

If the student who stutters is excused from oral classroom work, s/he may feel momentary relief, but the next time s/he faces such a situation, the fear and anxiety may be even greater.

We all feel better once we face a feared situation, and the student who stutters is no exception. When you speak to him/her, explain that excusing him/her from oral assignments won't help, because eventually, s/he will have to learn to speak to a group.

To make things **easier,** you might suggest some of the following:

1. The use of a slide or overhead projector for the presentation of material. (The student may feel more relaxed and stutter less if the class is not looking directly at him/her.)

2. Tape record part of the presentation. (People who stutter are usually more fluent when they talk with one person, or speak into a tape recorder in the privacy of their own home.)

3. Arrange for the student to meet with you two or three times before the presentation day for rehearsal. Once s/he knows you are on his/her side, anxiety will lessen.

4. Students with severe stuttering problems might be given the opportunity to do the first few oral presentations privately in front of the teacher, the next few in front of a small group, and gradually working up to presenting in front of the entire class.

Should I discuss the stuttering problem with the student's other teachers?

It is important that the rest of the staff (especially those involved with the student and the guidance department) be made aware of the problem. Help everyone to realize how this speech problem might affect the student's work in their class.

Can the child's stuttering be overcome?

Studies show that approximately one-half of all children who stutter become fluent. (However, the probability of this decreases with each passing year that the school-aged child stutters.) Some children improve significantly with treatment. We generally do not speak of a *cure* for stuttering. Our claims are to increase fluency, build self-confidence, help to reduce communication stress in the environment and help the student to accept him/herself.

Sometimes the student's speech is very fluent, and other times it is quite severe – why does it change?

A dysfluent child's speech will probably deteriorate when the child is tired, anxious, worried or uncertain.

The amount and severity of stuttering is affected by the situation and the alert teacher can help structure the school environment so that the student will encounter more success than failure. For example, avoid asking questions on a day when s/he is having a great deal of difficulty speaking, but do capitalize on a good day. The student's confidence will increase as s/he experiences more fluency.

[I recall being asked how to determine a good speech day from a bad one by more than one teacher. Some could not notice the fluctuation in my son's stutter which could go from mild to severe from one day to the next. To this question, I would always suggest to ask Lucas. He's never had a problem showing anyone that his throat is in a squeeze, provided it's done discreetly. If he's having a good day, he would simply say "Fire away!"]

Since much of the French Immersion Program is oral, how can I grade a student who stutters and is very hesitant to speak?

Students who stutter have difficulty in any activity which involves speaking to a group. Imagine how much more difficult it must be to try and speak in a language which is unfamiliar in both vocabulary and syntax.

Encourage the student to speak in class, and ask questions that you know s/he knows. If by the end of the term, you are unsure of his/her ability, speak to him/her privately for a half hour or so to assess his/her skills. If you still feel that the student might have more facility than s/he is able to show you, tape record questions and set a reasonable time limit for him/her to record the answers.

Remember that stuttering is a speaking problem, not a learning problem.

Anxiety, fear and tension may work together to prevent the student from expressing what s/he knows.

How can I prevent the rest of the class from laughing or teasing the student who stutters?

Often, very young children don't take too much notice of differences between themselves and their peers. By grade one, however, there may be problems with teasing and imitating. Some teachers have introduced the topic of individual differences to the class. They have asked each student and themselves, to reveal a trait or habit which makes him/her different from the others. Emphasize the idea that we are all different and that these differences make us more, and not less, valuable.

If the student is clearly upset by teasing, speak to him/her privately – at a time when s/he will not feel s/he is being punished (e.g., don't keep the student in at recess for a chat).

Tell the student that you know s/he is having difficulty with certain people in the class. Help him/her identify those few who are teasing and also help the student recognize that most of the class is on his/her side. Let the student know that you are available for more talks, if s/he wishes. Assure the student that you don't regard his/her speech as a problem and that you are really interested in what s/he has to say.

To increase self-confidence, consider making the student your helper. Maximize and praise his/her skills and achievements – be it in Math or simply his/her neatness.

Teasing may be a very difficult problem and one which is not easily solved in the upper grades. It will depend a great deal on the personality of the student. Probably the most helpful and positive move would be for the student to speak to the class about the problem. Most children respond sensitively when a problem is discussed openly and many speech-language pathologists encourage students to discuss their stuttering openly with their peers.

A classroom discussion of individual differences with personal input from everyone may also prove beneficial in the intermediate and senior grades.

A child is being seen for stuttering therapy: what can I do to help?

Speech-language pathologists are the professionals qualified to manage stuttering in children and adults. They work directly with the speech problem itself; help the student deal with his/her handicap and assist parents and teachers and all those involved with the student to understand and deal more effectively with the stuttering.

The speech-language pathologist normally contacts the classroom teacher to discuss the student's therapy program. The classroom teacher may be asked to help by documenting the student's daily speech behaviour using a simple checklist, or s/he might be asked to set aside a short time each day during which the child must make use of his speech techniques when responding to a question or when s/he is asked to read.

*   *   *

I include another article, *Stuttering in Young Children*, which was written by Paula Moss, B. Med. Sci. Hons. Speech of Ontario, Canada. I feel that this information would not only be beneficial to parents of young children who stutter, but also to the Nursery School and Kindergarten teachers directly involved with a dysfluent child.

In a recent letter I received from Paula, she mentioned she had been busy over the last twelve months, moving towards opening her own practice in Brampton, just outside of Toronto, Ontario. She added that as health services continue to be cut, speech is always one of the first to be marked non-essential, so her goal was to have her office set up by the end of March 1994, working alongside one of the local physicians.

> **Stuttering in Young Children . . .** Many children go through a period of hesitant or dysfluent speech in early childhood. Between the ages of 2 and 5 years of age, several will demonstrate varying degrees of difficulty producing smooth, fluent speech. This repeating, pausing and backing up of speech and the general confusion of "thinking and talking" is very normal as the child tries to master the most difficult skill he will ever learn, that of learning to talk.
>
> The amount and types of dysfluent behaviour can vary from one day to the next and across situations, sometimes with no apparent pattern. It often increases when the child is tired, excited, apprehensive or when he tries to compete with other speakers. Some children will outgrow this period of development, but some will not.
>
> Stuttering, if it continues into adolescence and adulthood, can be a crippling disorder, affecting the person's ability to communicate and socialize with others. It can have a significant impact on an individual's success at school, on job opportunities and on the ability to make friends. Indeed, it can be, and unfortunately often is, a very isolating disorder.
>
> For these reasons, early identification of and intervention for young children who stutter is crucial. When stuttering is detected early and remedial steps are taken, the results can be dramatic.
>
> Because it is often difficult to distinguish between normal dysfluencies and true stuttering, all professionals working with young children need to be aware of what constitutes a real problem. Children who are beginning to show true stuttering may also show differences in the frequency or amount and type of dysfluent behaviour. Seeking professional guidance in order to determine which children are at risk of long-term problems is crucial.

We learn from current research that physical, linguistic and situational factors can impact on the development and maintenance of stuttering. There is some evidence that people who stutter demonstrate some small differences in the way their speech is timed and coordinated. Stuttering also seems to run in families and affects boys more often than girls.

Learning and using language is a very complex process. Certain language forms are more likely to produce dysfluent speech. This would include longer sentences, complex sentences and questions and new unfamiliar words. A rapid speech rate will also impact on the ability to produce smooth speech.

Other factors that may interrupt the flow of speech include: being interrupted when speaking, being asked too many questions and short pause times between turns in the conversation. Also important is the reaction of others to the stuttering behaviour. Responding negatively to the child can aggravate the problem.

Children vary widely in the number and type of dysfluent behaviour, but it is possible to differentiate between normal dysfluencies and stuttering. The following are examples of normal dysfluencies:

1. whole word and phrase repetitions: "My my mommy is coming" or "I want, I want a cookie;" and

2. pauses filled with "um" or "er" – "I, er want a cookie."

Typically, the dysfluent behaviour is produced easily without struggle and accounts for less than 5% of the child's speech.

The following behaviours may be a sign that the child is more at risk:

1. part-word repetitions: "B-b-b-because I want to";

2. stretching of sounds: "Caaaan I do it"; and

3. struggle behaviours including facial grimacing, rapid eye blinks, head or jaw movements and irregular breathing.

Other warning signs include, if the stuttering behaviour accounts for more than 5% of the child's speech, if it is getting worse or if the child appears to be embarrassed by his speech.

What you can do to help:

1. Slow down the rate of speech and the conversational pace when talking with young children. Children often try to match the speech rate of those around them. If those rates are too fast for the child's motor skill, the fluency may break down.

2. Simplify grammar and vocabulary and use shorter sentences. Long, complex sentences may stress the child's processing system. Children may also attempt to copy these sentences and may not have the competence to do so.

3. Reduce the use of direct questions. Questions place significant demands on fluency and prompt a child to process the question, form a response and answer quickly. Often, if the child does not answer quickly, we fire another question, thus causing an interruption and confusion.

4. Reduce interruptions and increase wait time. Children need to know that they have lots of time to think and talk. They need to know that others are listening to them. Interruptions will frustrate them and increase dysfluent behaviour.

5. It is NOT a good idea to tell them to slow down, to stop and start again or take a big breath before they talk. Instead, we will make children more aware that there is something wrong with the way they talk. They may start to feel worried about their speech and even avoid talking in some situations.

As good communication skills are essential to success in all areas of development, it is vital that the stuttering child be assessed as soon as the problem is suspected. A visit to a qualified speech-language pathologist would give a child who stutters the best possible start in life.

*   *   *

Some people who stutter or parents of children who stutter may wish to consider other therapy approaches such as the use of various devices worn on the body to help the individual achieve and maintain fluency outside the clinic. Among the most popular fluency aids are: the Vocal Feedback Device, Brand Name: Vocaltech Clinical Vocal Feedback Device; the Aural Enhancement of Vocal Tone, Brand Name: Fluency Master; the Electronic Metronome, Brand Name: Pace Master and the Electronic Masker, Brand Name: Edinburgh Masker.

In a 1993 article published in her own newsletter *The Staff*, Janice Westbrook, Ph.D., CCC-SP of Garland, Texas, U.S.A. recommended that parents ask the following important questions with regard to fluency aids:

1. Can the device be used with assurance that my child will not be physically harmed in any way, over a brief or extended period of time?

2. Will my child learn new skills from using the device?

3. Will fluency attained by using the device transfer to other situations, or should we expect that our child will need the device indefinitely?

4. Will use of the device promote my child's sense of independence?

5. What were the results of short-term and long-term research studies investigating this device?

6. Will this device be convenient, attractive and unobtrusive as my child uses it outside of therapy?

7. How expensive is the device to produce, and what profit is being made on its distribution?

8. Will insurance coverage be provided for this device?

*   *   *

Although the apparent hope is that these devices will function as well as the hearing aid, parents interested in this form of intervention are advised to proceed with caution.

CHAPTER 8

CREATING GREATER AWARENESS

From mid to late 1991, I started working on a special project. It had occurred to me that as an organized group, parents could accomplish much more on behalf of children who stutter. Actually, the idea had been suggested to me more than a year earlier when William G. Webster, Ph.D., then Professor of Psychology at Carleton University of Ottawa, Canada, wrote me a letter to comment on some of the materials I had written about Lucas.

Dr. Webster is the author of the recently published *Facilitating Fluency: Transfer Strategies for Adult Stuttering Treatment Programs*, a client manual he co-wrote with the late Marie Poulos. In addition to this manual, William Webster has done extensive research on stuttering, and continues to do so in his new position at Brock University in St. Catharines, Ontario. In his August 9, 1990, letter, Dr. Webster wrote:

> I think there may be a real place for a self-help group for parents of children who stutter. Such a group could provide information about stuttering both to parents and children, provide an opportunity for an exchange of experiences about managing stuttering in children, and develop a political and public education arm to effect some change in how children who stutter are dealt with in schools, and in providing better treatment opportunities for children.
>
> It seems to me that through your writing you have shown the potential to lead the formation of such a group, and I would encourage you to do so. There continues to be much ignorance about stuttering and, equally, a lot of misdirected parental guilt (and misdirected blame by teachers) that goes back to outdated and discredited ideas about the psychological origins of stuttering. A parent group could do a great deal to dispel these myths and help families deal realistically with stuttering in their children.

*   *   *

With this kind of encouragement, one would think I could move quickly towards my goal of creating greater awareness for stuttering. It was not the case; I didn't know where to start. Seeing that local hospitals and school board speech and language departments were not at liberty to hand over their lists of patients to me, I had to find another way to reach parents like me. I sent notices to all local schools and school boards, churches, recreational facilities, shopping malls, medical centres, dental clinics and any other place I could think of. What brought me the most response, however, was a Letter to the Editor which was published simultaneously from August 1991 to early January 1992 in 22 local and area newspapers. It read like this:

> My son is disabled. He stutters. For some of you who may not know, stuttering involves various speech difficulties often accompanied by typical behavioral patterns not easily identified by teachers and school authorities. Lack of knowledge about this communication difficulty can result in a variety of unpleasant experiences for dysfluent children.
>
> Stuttering is not something a child does on purpose, nor is it something he does because he has been psychologically traumatized at a younger age. Although this explanation may work for other disorders observed in children, all current medical journals support the view that stuttering is a neurologically-based handicap which can affect speech and behaviour. Any type of stressful situation, however, can have a drastic effect on a child's ability to control his stutter.
>
> I firmly believe that a proactive approach to stuttering could alleviate a lot of misunderstanding surrounding this communication disorder. It is imperative that all educators learn more about stuttering and simple methods to help the stuttering child communicate effectively in the classroom setting. Unfortunately, documentation on stuttering is practically non-existent in our school systems which makes it doubly difficult for teachers to help children afflicted with this ailment.
>
> I know there are a lot of other parents of children who stutter in the Ottawa area. As a group, we can make school boards react to the urgency of implementing various strategies to help our children who are working so hard to be understood by others.
>
> If you have a child who stutters, please attend our first meeting to be held on January 16, 1992, 7:30 PM at the Rehabilitation Centre in Ottawa, Ontario.

*   *   *

The response to this article was gratifying. Dozens of calls were made to my home and many parents confirmed their attendance. Thanks to my good friend John Ahlbach of San Francisco, I had an adequate supply of *Teacher Tips* brochures and other informative materials on stuttering for distribution to my newly-formed local parent group. Noticing the excitement in my voice when we talked on the telephone, John warned me to start thinking in terms of a smaller turnout.

Having worked hard at getting the attention of parents of children who stutter, fluency specialists and educators for several months, I must admit that I envisioned hundreds of people in attendance at my first parents' meeting. John was cautious not to rain on my parade, but he did manage to bring me back to reality. "If you get just one or two parents, you will have done beautifully," he said, "focus on helping them. Sooner or later, you will reach others, but for the time being, you must anticipate that almost anything that has to do with stuttering does not attract a lot of people."

A major storm had been brewing outside for most of the day on January 16, 1992. At the rate the snow was blowing, I doubted anyone at all would be able to make it. However, in spite of the storm, seven parents and the Chief of Psychological Services from one of our local school boards was present. We had a good meeting which lasted over two hours. The next day, I received telephone calls from eight other parents who wanted to be there, but couldn't because of the storm.

In the months that followed, I started to get calls from parents from all over the province of Ontario. It seemed almost inevitable that I would move on to organizing a provincial group instead of keeping it at the local level only. Thus, the *Ontario Stuttering Project (OSP)* was formed. I started to prepare notices for distribution across the province, informing parents, individual teachers, all Ontario School Boards and speech-language pathologists of the upcoming one-day speech conference scheduled for April 11, 1992. It was held in Ottawa at the Rehabilitation Centre where I was once again granted access to a conference room thanks to the help provided by Sue Carroll-Thomas, Director of the Communication Disorders Department.

My first speech conference had been planned for April instead of March when we Ottawans still run the risk of a snow storm. My heart sank when I opened the door to a foot of snow the morning of the conference. We never get snow in April! Well, almost never.

Luckily, all 60 people who had confirmed their attendance made it to the event safely. They had travelled from all over Ontario; some came from Stayner, Thornbury, Toronto and L'Orignal. One parent and her son had travelled 15 hours by bus from Hearst; others came from Arnprior, Aylmer (Quebec), Orleans, Vanier, Nepean and naturally, several were from Ottawa. The mere fact that the unexpected storm did not deter anyone from coming said a lot about my parent members. The event was a great success followed by a pyjama party at my house for four, or was it five?? of the young participants at the conference.

Thanks to the generous sponsorship I obtained from my friends, the *Ontario Barber Shop Singers*, I was able to start producing a bi-monthly newsletter I called *On Target*. It was the only way I could think of to keep everyone posted on my progress. Continued support from George Shields, Chairman of the *Harmonize for Speech Fund* of the Ontario Barber Shop Singers, enabled me to produce, print and distribute eleven issues over the two-year period which followed.

The newsletter contained helpful material for use in our Ontario schools; it became a vehicle through which parents could voice their concerns about their children's stuttering and the lack of treatment possibilities in many communities. What I liked the most about *On Target* was the *Kids Corner* section where children had the opportunity to talk about their stuttering and to connect with other children who have the same problem.

Throughout the years, my son had often felt so alone. He was, and remains the only student with this speech problem in all five schools he has attended so far. When he was younger, Lucas looked forward to receiving the U.S. newsletter called *The Staff* which contained letters written by other children who stuttered (see Chapter Ten for more information about this newsletter).

From the heart of children who stutter were written the following words for publication in *On Target*:

Sometimes my stuttering makes me wish I never had speech problems . . .

My stuttering sometimes embarrasses me in front of my friends . . .

Sometimes I feel sad when I stutter because the kids tease me. My stutters gets very bad when I get excited and when I am asked a lot of questions. To get back on track, I practice my breathing. I am glad that you care about us enough to organize a group . . .

Having a speech problem can be hard, but you have to be tough and stand up for yourself. It's good to have a friend to help you at times. Dealing with my speech is hard. When new kids come to my class, I feel shy so I don't talk around them, or I just talk to them when I have to, for example, "do you want to be on my soccer team." I take out my anger on skiing and basketball. Kids in my class don't tease me because they don't mind, and if they do, they will get a pounding!

PICTURE THIS . . . This scene is all too familiar to all children who stutter. A teacher asks them a question, and no matter if they know it or not, they take the easy way out so they don't have to stutter in front of their friends. Then the bullies of the class laugh at them and tease them because they can't talk like everyone else.

When your teacher is at the front of the class asking questions to all your friends, you are hoping he won't ask you. But he does, and you feel yourself start to get flustered and start to sweat, your brain is racing, your heart is beating faster and faster with every second. The teacher asks the question, and you know the answer so you try to speak, but you stutter. All of the class starts to laugh at you. You feel like you just want to run away. But it really doesn't matter if you stutter because everybody is the same on the inside and we all have our good points.

My stuttering makes my throat tight, like it's squeezing together. It makes me feel like a person from another planet. It helps when I relax my breathing.

Stuttering doesn't hurt because people who stutter are special. I think speech therapy helps my speech a lot. In my school, whenever my teacher asks us to read, I get nervous and skip ahead to see if there are words that I will stutter on. I'm happy that I have some friends who stutter like me . . .

*   *   *

Not only did I receive great articles for publication in my newsletter, but there were many creative drawings, all of which I considered to be very special. This Chapter would not be complete without the inclusion of these drawings.

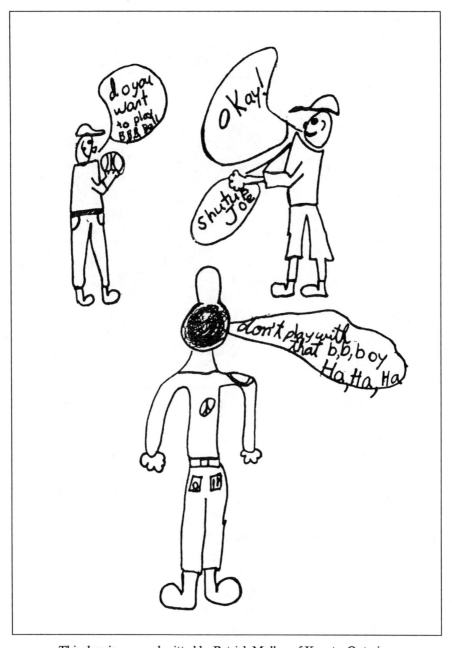

This drawing was submitted by Patrick Mullen of Kanata, Ontario.

* * *

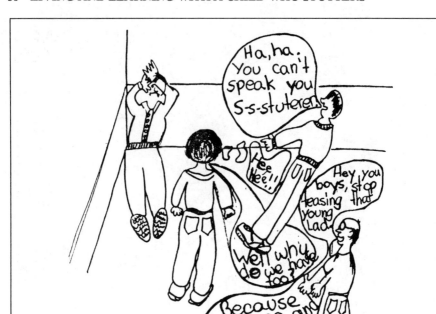

Patrick Mullen's sister Stephanie submitted her own special drawing.

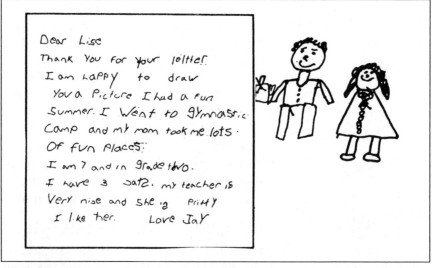

One of several happy pictures I received from Jay McCague of Cookstown, Ontario

STUTTERING
A comic strip.

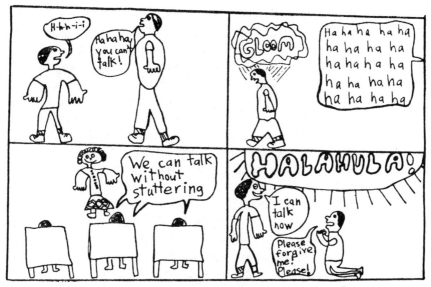

Scott Greenhorn of L'Orignal, Ontario, provided me with an excellent cover picture for the very popular September-October 1992 *On Target* issue.

Organizing the OSP enabled me to reach out to many parents and children, and it also gave me the opportunity to meet and talk to some very interesting people. Among them was Douglas H. Fullerton, O.C., M.Com., LL.D., D.U.C.

Born in St. John's, Newfoundland on September 3, 1917, Mr. Fullerton has had many successes throughout his career in spite of his stutter. He is the author of *The Capital of Canada: How should it be Governed?* 1974, *The Dangerous Delusion: Quebec's Independence Obsession,* 1978, *Graham Towers and his Times, a Biography of the 1st Governor of the Bank of Canada,* 1986. His most visible accomplishment, however, is the Rideau Canal skating rink, the world's longest, which got its start during his tenure as Chairman of Canada's National Capital Commission from 1969 to 1973.

I called Mr. Fullerton shortly after our local newspaper had done an excellent feature on him and his numerous achievements. I told him about the organization I had formed, and asked him if he would be interested in submitting a short article for publication in my newsletter. He asked that I send him a copy of *On Target* so he could get a better feel for the piece he agreed to write.

Two days later, I received a telephone call from Mr. Fullerton who seemed genuinely impressed with the edition I had forwarded to him. That particular edition included an article written by Jock Carlisle, Ph.D., someone he knew. Jokingly, he added he could write a much better article than Dr. Carlisle's, and if I happened to be talking to Jock in the near future, he wanted me to tell him so. Interestingly enough, Douglas Fullerton had written a review of Jock Carlisle's book *Tangled Tongue* which was published in our local paper back in 1985, a review that sent me rushing to the nearest bookstore to purchase a copy.

As I maintained contact with Dr. Carlisle and his wife Joan since we met at Lucas' refresher course, I sent Jock a short note telling him Douglas Fullerton was out to top his article. "Let him try!" said Jock who had been amused by Douglas' comment.

Shortly after, I was invited to Mr. Fullerton's house to pick up the article he had completed for my newsletter. We had an interesting talk during which he told me that what he had found most frustrating about stuttering was that people always paid too much attention to the way the communication was made rather than listen to WHAT was said. He added that he had prepared and delivered many speeches in his lifetime, after which comments would be made on his courage instead of focusing on the message or the purpose of his discussion.

Then he gave me a copy of a paper he had presented to the Special Parliamentary Committee on the Disabled and the Handicapped. Although Mr. Fullerton's submission on stuttering dates back to September 17, 1980, you will probably be as surprised as I to note that all of the issues raised in this document are applicable to today's situation with regard to stuttering. Obviously, our Canadian Government has not yet addressed any of the important points made by Mr. Fullerton in his submission; if it had, I probably would not have written this book. I would like to share Douglas Fullerton's words which were made public almost fourteen years ago.

Submission on Stuttering by Douglas H. Fullerton, September 17, 1980 . . . I have no mandate to speak for Canada's quarter million stutterers, other than that derived from my sixty years as a stutterer, and from the fact that I have survived it. We stutterers have never banded together as an organized group to lobby government aid for our particular handicap; the nature of our ailment is such as to almost compel us to go our individual way in silence. It is not the kind of ailment, either, which produces a Terry Fox.

Yet something has to be put before you about this strangely disabling and little understood disorder, if only because it is a serious handicap for so many people, and because in spite of the thousands of years of mankind's experience with stuttering, we have made little progress in finding its cause or discovering a cure. It is not accidental, by the way, that the word cure is seldom used by speech therapists; they have learned to suggest rather that the stutterer will be helped, or improved.

Several recent books have done a commendable job of bringing together many of the myths, facts and theories about stuttering, including a short book by Gerald Jonas,* a writer and former stutterer. His sub-title fairly describes the ailments: "The Disorder of Many Theories," for stuttering remains today one of the great mysteries of medicine. Certainly, the medical profession has played little part in advancing understanding of the ailment, and the doctors themselves have just about contracted out of treating it. Most of them are relieved to refer the patient to speech therapy, usually without knowing much about it.

Thus the stutterer seeking help will usually end up in one of two places: in larger cities where there is likely to be a speech clinic at a hospital, or, in the case of children, a speech therapist in school. The form of treatment will often depend on the training received by the therapist, which varies widely. Alternatively, the stutterer (males outnumber females 4:1) may answer an advertisement of a cured stutterer who hangs out his shingle as a therapist; here the variation of qualifications and methods is even wider, and complicated by the existence of a number of quacks whose main motivation is profit.

It must be noted that there are easier ways of making a living, because the treatment of stuttering is a slow, discouraging business which normally depends on an unusual degree of dedication on the part of the therapist. And, although permanent cures are few, almost any form of treatment that forces the stutterer to focus on his problem does have therapeutic value, at least over the short term). What is lacking in all the approaches, however, is the common denominator of agreement on the best approach to treatment, or even a generally accepted theory of the cause(s) of stuttering.

I can't begin to cover in this paper the various hypotheses about causes, or discuss the merits of various forms of treatment, partly because I don't feel qualified to do so. My contact with stuttering has rather been through personal experience, curiosity or discussions with therapists. My purpose, rather, is to make these points:

1. stuttering is indeed a serious emotional, social and economic handicap to those who suffer from it, and needs wider recognition as such;

2. current treatment rests on a non-solid foundation of knowledge or research, but is rather a grab-bag of older methods, laced with a few modern theories or technical gimmicks (although almost any treatment is better than none); and

3. the principal need of the stutterer is for access to treatment that works for him. The availability of such help, however, presupposes a much greater application of resources to a renewed search into the origins or cause(s) of the ailment, and into the best way of approaching it therapeutically.

Let me elaborate briefly on these points. Some progress has been made in recent years in recognizing the disabling nature of stuttering. I was heartened to see an editorial in *The Globe and Mail* a few months ago which described it as a terrible handicap, preventing the full use of a faculty that in our society is all but indispensable. The editorial was provoked by cuts in Ontario's health budgets which denied many stutterers access to treatment (the newspaper should not be faulted for its unawareness of the inadequacies in existing treatment). Certainly, as Jonas pointed out, the ability to communicate through language defines us as human beings in a society. Milton's poetic reference to his blindness could aptly be applied to stutterers,

And that one talent which is death to hide
Lodged with me useless . . .

Yet there are other dimensions to it, as I can personally attest. One is the dilemma of all stutterers that they can never really be reconciled to accepting their disability because of their intermittent periods of fluency. There are, of course, handicaps more disabling than stuttering, but in almost all of them, such as blindness, the afflicted person at some stage usually comes to accept his condition, and builds his life accordingly.

The stutterer becomes so skilled at adapting his speech to try to avoid feared sounds that the avoidance process eventually becomes almost automatic and uncontrollable: the spasms may be less frequent, but the meaning often gets lost in the shuffle. A tape of a stutterer's speech shows how tortuous the process can become. In giving a speech, I have found it difficult – usually impossible – to follow a prepared text.

The emotionally damaging part of stuttering cuts across a gamut of human feelings: embarrassment at being seen to stutter, a sense of inferiority or rejection, anticipatory fear of the spasms themselves, panic during the spasm, guilt or shame at failure or backsliding in treatment, and, perhaps worst of all, frustration at being unable to communicate one's thoughts adequately to others.

This last is a particular problem for adult stutterers, and certainly for me is the most serious aspect of my own stutter. When I speak, the words seldom come out as my mind dictates – the semi-automatic form of spasm-evasion takes over, arguments are presented in truncated form, words are dropped or swallowed in haste to get finished, nuances or qualifying phrases tend to get lost. **It is on the way the words come out, however, that the stutterer's competence or intelligence tend to be measured.**

It almost goes without saying that no stutterer can perform at his maximum capacity, although there may be compensations in some form, as there are with most handicaps. Yet job performance is affected, access to many professions is denied, and the emotional fall-out from the daily trauma of speech forces many stutterers in effect to hide from the world - to seek low level occupations where no speech demands are made upon them. What the totality of the economic cost to Canadian society is, I cannot guess, but it is great.

The second concern I raise is about the quality of present treatment. I am no authority of current techniques, but I have read a bit about them and spoken to a number of speech therapists, and the approach still appears to be based essentially on traditional techniques – slowing the pace of speech, keeping air flowing between syllables, conditioning the stutterer to feared situations by deliberate exposure to them, reducing the severity of spasm, etc.. The only new approaches seem to be those based on electronic technology, such as delayed auditory feedback, or hidden electronic metronomes, which set the pace of speech at a level at which the stutterer feels comfortable, and can be reasonably fluent.

I have noted that almost anything the stutterer does to focus on his speech problem – really to face his problem – tends to be at least of short-run benefit. Existing approaches to treatment have this in common:

1. they are pragmatic or experimental, and based on non-agreed explanations for the cause(s) of the ailment; no one could quarrel with an approach that worked, but the rate of permanent success of all of them is low, and

2. the amount of scientific research into the treatment and cause(s) of stuttering is negligible, and generally carried out by those who stutter themselves or become accidentally involved.

3. In this search, the medical profession has not been prominent. Government involvement has essentially been to agree on the need for therapy, provide some funds for this purpose, but to make little attempt to determine the qualifications of the therapists, or whether the methods or results are good, bad or indifferent.

In a society which increasingly is concerned about looking after the deprived, the disabled and the handicapped, this state of affairs should no longer be allowed to continue. What I suggest your Committee can do is this:

1. First, recognize publicly that the ailment is a handicap for the 1%, more or less, of adult Canadians who stutter (and 5% of children), that research and treatment are inadequate and not very scientific, and that governments and the medical profession should do something about it.

2. Second, since ignorance about the ailment is so widespread, propose a task force or commission to review the present state of knowledge about stuttering and methods of treatment, and to provide a forum for public and medical discussion. (One place to begin would be to review what Canadian medical schools teach, if anything, about stuttering, and how hospital clinics are treating it.) And because stuttering is an almost universal ailment, we may well have something to learn from other countries about it.

3. Finally, I assume one of your principal goals is to discover and throw light on job discrimination against the handicapped.

Stutterers are certainly handicapped in the work place, but I have difficulty in seeing how affirmative action on their behalf could be enforced. Stuttering is an impediment in areas involving oral communication, closing off many jobs to stutterers. What might be of some help is to provide some tribunal to which the stutterer could appeal against what he feels to be unjust treatment that arises solely because of his ailment.

* Gerald Jonas: *Stuttering*, Noonday Press, New York, 1977.

* * *

In January 1994, it was with great regret that I informed OSP members of my plans to discontinue the publication of my newsletter and the many other activities I had taken on over the past three years. It was a tough decision to make, one with which I still don't feel completely comfortable, but I was left with no other alternative. These hard economic times we live in made it impossible to obtain sufficient financial support from government, corporate and private sources. Given the difficulties experienced by established charities as they try to remain in operation with budgets which keep getting smaller every year, I had to face the reality that the formation of a new charitable organization would be even more risky.

I'm hopeful that Canada will eventually be successful at establishing a country-wide support network for adults and children who stutter. Over the last four years, CAPS, the Canadian Association for People who Stutter has made great progress in that direction. There have been two well attended speech conferences so far; the first was held in Banff, Alberta, and the second took place in my Ottawa home town just two summers ago. Plans for a third conference in Toronto have been underway for some time. This third national speech conference to be held in the summer of 1995, will probably bring about more positive changes for those who stutter, their families, friends and significant others. For more information on this organization, see the CAPS listing in Reference Guide.

CHAPTER 9

LEARNING TO LIVE FOR THE MOMENT

I don't think there has ever been a day when I could pretend Lucas' stuttering did not exist. It continues to impact our life and his, but certainly to a much lesser degree since his enrolment at a school where he was given the opportunity to be himself without having to worry about anyone's reaction to his handicap. It made all the difference on his outlook on life and all it has to offer him.

Although there has been a dramatic change in Lucas' reaction to the sound of the telephone ringing, I had learned to accept that he would not pick it up when it rang, even though he would be standing right next to it. There were times when I found that particularly exasperating, especially when I was in the midst of baking a batch of cookies or scrubbing a dirty pot, but I would rinse my hands, step over to the kitchen wall phone, and ask Lucas to kindly step aside while I answered the call.

It would make my day when the phone call happened to be from one of his friends, and Lucas would roll his eyes and say: "How was I supposed to know it would be for me!" Nowadays, our teenager jumps on the telephone before anyone else has a chance to pick it up. He doesn't want me to find out how many girlfriends he is dating at the same time! He has also become a real chatterbox on the phone; he can go on for hours at a time, to the extent that the rest of us have to beg him to get off the line when we need to make a call of our own. I realize we are in a no-win situation here in that both telephone scenarios are equally inconvenient. Thank goodness for call waiting.

When the boys were younger, dinner time was somewhat awkward. We would all make an effort to be as patient as possible when Lucas spoke at the supper table. I would have to make sure he got equal time to speak even though his brother was dying to interrupt. If he was interrupted, there would be more facial grimacing and blockages after which he would almost always give up. In addition, I would slow down the rate of my own speech so he could take his cue from me to make better use of his speech targets.

Our dinner hour then seemed to take all the fun out of eating and talking about each other's day. Family dinners are now a rarity as all four of us are on different schedules. Things like hockey games, basketball practice and hanging out with friends at the mall have a tendency to interfere with my meal planning. I make time to prepare an excellent supper for four and nobody shows up, or I get: "I'll eat later, Mom." Some days when I get carried away with my work and forget about cooking, Lucas will come home from school with a couple of his buddies, all three in a ravenous state. Kraft dinner, coming right up!

Whereas he needed constant coaxing to go out and be with people he had never met, he goes just about anywhere now. This week he came home with a job application he had picked up at a shoe store. My husband and I wondered how he managed to ask for it, however, he came home with it so he obviously hadn't shied away from a new speaking situation.

He enjoys going to new places with his friends and has the self-confidence to deal with the speech difficulties on his own. He's very open about his feelings. Just a couple of weekends ago, he said he wouldn't be caught dead being seen with us at a movie theatre! I suppose we had it coming and should have known better to ask if he would like to join us now that he's at the tender – or is it touchy-age of fifteen.

Even though we have all learned not to focus of Lucas' stuttering, it will continue to be a part of our everyday life as a family. It can't be helped, but I think the special bond we have developed over the years has made the difference in my son's ability to cope with his handicap.

He started high school last September and it was difficult for him to adjust to the new school setting. Although I am confident that my eldest son Jonathan has the potential and the determination to achieve whatever goals he sets out for himself, I often wonder what the future holds for Lucas as I feel that society isn't quite ready for people who stutter. Will the demands on his speech be too great for him to complete high school? What about college? I can't see myself requesting a parent/teacher conference to discuss Lucas' stuttering with college or university professors. Will he go after the job he really wants in spite of his speech problem, or will he settle for something else?

Perhaps none of these questions really matter because in my heart, I know I have been successful at making him feel good about himself. His sensitivity, his magnetic personality, his wit and his compassion for others are just a few of his many qualities which will bring him closer to freedom of speech.

CHAPTER 10

STUTTERING, THE BRAIN, AND EMOTIONS

by David Forster, M.Sc.

I have been asked to add a few words to this book about the state of scientific evidence on the cause of stuttering. That is really a very large topic; there are many different theories about what causes stuttering, and I am by no means an expert on all of them. I have chosen instead to try to give you a general flavour of the kind of research that has been done on stuttering, but to focus on the theory I know the most about.

For a long time there have been two essentially opposing viewpoints about the cause of stuttering. On the one hand, there are those who regard stuttering as a "psychological" disorder. On the other hand, there are those who consider stuttering to be a biological or physiological disorder based in the brain.

There are many "psychological" theories about stuttering. For example, Prof. W. Johnson argued in the 1950's that the onset of stuttering in a child is related to the actions of the child's parents. It is now widely accepted that there is virtually *no* scientific evidence to support such an idea. A child's stuttering is not the fault of his or her parents.

Stuttering has also been described as a learned disorder, an emotional disorder, a neurotic disorder and a psychosexual disorder, among others. However, it is probably safe to say that the majority of speech scientists and speech pathologists today would view stuttering, at its core, as a physiological disorder based in the brain. That doesn't mean that there aren't psychological aspects of stuttering. There certainly are, and they can affect the individual's life in a significant way. But they are secondary to the biological basis of stuttering. That biological predisposition comes first. The psychological characteristics then follow.

In a way, the rift between those who see stuttering as "psychological" and those who see it as "biological" is unfortunate. Regardless of its root cause, both biological and psychological factors are involved in the expression of stuttering in the individual from moment to moment and situation to situation. We cannot truly understand the neurological basis of stuttering if we ignore the psychological factors that influence its expression. We must be interested in the relationship between the psychology and the neurology of stuttering. In the coming sections, I will attempt to do just that. First, however, I will address the biological aspect of stuttering. Why do we think the root cause of stuttering is "biological" rather than "psychological?"

A Biological Cause of Stuttering

Genetic Evidence

Stuttering runs in families. That alone does not prove a genetic cause, but it is a starting point. The *way* stuttering runs in families increases our confidence that there is a genetic cause to stuttering. Boys stutter more than girls (about a 2:1 ratio which increases with age as more girls than boys grow out of it). However, mothers are more likely to transmit stuttering to their children than fathers. So the son of a mother who stutters is the most likely to develop stuttering, while the daughter of a father who stutters is much less likely to develop stuttering. Of course, children with no parents who stutter are the least likely to develop stuttering.

Perhaps the best evidence of a genetic component to stuttering is from twin studies conducted by Pauline Howie. In one study she compared "monozygotic" (identical) twins to "dizygotic" (non-identical) twins. Monozygotic twins are identical genetically. Dizygotic twins are no more similar genetically than any two siblings. Dr. Howie found that if one identical twin stutters, the other will also stutter 73% of the time. However, if one non-identical twin stutters, the other will stutter only 32% of the time. The difference in the "agreement" rates between identical and non-identical twins strongly suggests that there is a genetic cause to stuttering.

Of course, it is likely that genetic factors are not the whole story. If they were, then if one identical twin stuttered, the other would also stutter 100% of the time. The fact that one identical twin stutters and the other doesn't does not mean that genetics are not involved, however. To illustrate this point, I will refer to a different condition that has a genetic cause: harelip. A harelip is a physical abnormality of the upper lip, and has a well-known genetic cause. However, it is possible for one identical twin to have a harelip while the other one does not. Geneticists would call this an "incompletely penetrant" genetic trait. Some people with a given gene will have the condition, others won't. In the case of stuttering, it may be that environmental circumstances which we do not yet understand can influence whether or not the individual will stutter.

Neuropsychological Evidence

What do "neuropsychologists" do? Before discussing neuropsychological research on stuttering, I will briefly describe what neuropsychology is and what neuropsychologists do. A neuropsychologist is a unique kind of psychologist who uses his or her knowledge of the relationship between brain and behaviour to make educated guesses about what is happening in somebody's brain. Neuropsychologists generally rely on *behaviour* to draw their conclusions about the brain. They will use their knowledge of the brain and behaviour to devise clever tests involving motor skills, perceptual skills, or cognitive skills that can reveal important information about the functioning of a person's brain. There are a variety of such tests that suggest that there are subtle differences between the brains of people who stutter and fluent speakers.

Activity in the Two Cerebral Hemispheres: Many people know that the most advanced part of the human brain, the cerebrum, is divided into two halves. These halves are called the "cerebral hemispheres." In most people, speech and language are controlled mostly by the left hemisphere, while emotions and "spatial skills" (e.g. the ability to recognize complex shapes) are controlled to a greater extent by the right hemisphere. There are other cognitive abilities that are controlled mostly by one or the other hemisphere as well. Early in this century two very eminent scholars, Lee Travis and Samuel Orton, proposed that people who stutter have speech centres in both cerebral hemispheres instead of just the left one. They thought that the signals from the two sides of the brain were "competing" for control of the speech muscles, and that this was what caused stuttering. In support of this idea they pointed to evidence at the time that left-handers and forced right-handers were more likely to stutter than pure right-handers. Travis also conducted experiments where he measured the electrical impulses arriving at the two sides of the jaw. He found that the impulses arriving at the two sides weren't synchronized as well in his subjects who stuttered as they were in fluent speakers.

In the past thirty years, neuropsychologists and other neuroscientists have been able to use more sophisticated tests to investigate whether or not Orton and Travis were correct. It is clear that, in a strict sense, they were not correct. People who stutter seem to have their speech centres in their left hemisphere, just like fluent speakers. Nevertheless, there may have been an element of truth in the ideas of Orton and Travis. There does appear to be something unusual about the relationship between the left and right hemispheres in people who stutter.

In our lab we have done some experiments to investigate this phenomenon, and we have reviewed the experiments other scientists have done. We believe that the difference between people who stutter and fluent speakers may involve the way they *use* their left and right hemispheres, rather than the actual makeup of the two hemispheres. Compared to fluent speakers, people who stutter seem to have more activity in their right hemisphere when they are engaged in speech and language-related tasks. The reason for this is unclear. Also, I must stress that it is a *difference*, and is not necessarily a weakness of any kind. In the coming sections, I will mention other evidence in support of this idea, and will describe how it might influence speech fluency.

Motor Control: There is also evidence of differences in the motor skills of people who stutter. Motor "coordination" is actually a poor term because it refers to a wide range of sensory, motor, and cognitive processes. There are many such abilities that may be controlled by completely different parts of the brain. In general, people who stutter are not uncoordinated. But there are certain very specific aspects of motor performance that appear to be mildly impaired in people who stutter. These are related to the timing of the many individual muscle groups that must work together to create a larger movement. For example, in speech, the muscles that make up the tongue, jaw, lips, cheeks, voicebox and diaphragm all must work together to create a precisely orchestrated series of movements. A very subtle difficulty with that timing might show up as a more substantial problem with creating fluent speech sounds.

This "timing problem" has been well-documented by speech scientists. But it is not specific to speech, and has been demonstrated in hand movements as well. It is a very mild problem, and may well be totally irrelevant to nonspeech movements. Keep in mind that there are professional athletes and musicians who stutter. Dave Taylor, the hockey player who had been so kind to Lucas, is by no means "uncoordinated." Speech is a task that requires the very precise timing of hundreds of little movements in rapid succession, and even tiny disruptions in that timing might cause it to break down. Similar tiny disruptions in the timing of hand movements would not be as serious, because subsequent movements can compensate for them.

Electrical Activity in the Two Cerebral Hemispheres

Some researchers have shown differences between people who stutter and fluent speakers in electrical brain activity. These studies use variations of the "electroencephalogram" or EEG. The EEG is a machine that measures the electrical activity in the brain through sensitive electrodes attached to the person's scalp. In general, people who stutter do not have "abnormal" EEG patterns. However, there are some subtle differences that one can demonstrate between a group of people who stutter and a group of fluent speakers. The most commonly reported difference is that people who stutter have more activity in the right side of their brain than fluent speakers when performing speech or language-related tasks. As you may have noted, this finding is in agreement with findings from neuropsychological experiments that I have already mentioned.

Brain Scans

Since the mid-1970s, a variety of powerful new techniques for looking at the brain in the living human have been developed. The first of these techniques, the CT scan and the MRI scan, look at the *structure* of the brain. They give a picture that looks like a slice through the brain. I am not aware of any evidence from CT or MRI studies of anatomical differences between the brains of people who stutter and fluent speakers.

However, a different class of brain scans (including "PET," "rCBF" and "SPECT" scans among others) has been developed even more recently. These truly marvelous scans actually show the *activity* of the brain. Like CT and MRI scans, they also show a "slice" of the brain, but instead of representing the anatomy, they use numbers or different colours to represent the amount of activity in different areas. Scans of this kind *have* shown differences between people who stutter and fluent speakers.

Some of these differences are specific to given tasks. For example, these scans also show more activity in the right hemisphere of people who stutter than in fluent speakers when they are involved in speech or language tasks. Note again that this is similar to the ideas discussed above with respect to neuropsychological and EEG studies.

However, even when the person is just asked to sit quietly and relax, there are differences between people who stutter and fluent speakers in other brain areas. What is perhaps most interesting is that these brain areas make sense in terms of what we know about stuttering and the neurology of speech. In particular, the evidence I mentioned above regarding the timing of muscular movements would lead us to suspect some of the very brain areas that have been implicated by those brain scans. One area we are especially interested in is the "Supplementary Motor Area" (SMA).

The SMA is very important for the timing of complex movements, including both speech and nonspeech (e.g. hand) movements. It is especially important in the planning stages of the movement. A problem in the SMA would show up as a difficulty in the initiation of movements. As you can probably see, this makes sense in the context of stuttering.

Do People Who Stutter Have "Brain Damage?"

As far as we know today, the answer is an emphatic no. That doesn't mean that there isn't a very mild form of damage at the microscopic level that we haven't seen yet. Everyone has a certain number of tiny spots in their brain where the normal arrangement of brain cells got "messed up" during development (these are called "cytoarchitectonic abnormalities)." It has been shown that people with severe dyslexia, for example, have a few more of these tiny abnormalities than is normally the case, and that they are clustered around certain areas of the brain. It is at least possible that something similar may be involved in some cases of stuttering; the research (which requires microscopic post-mortem examination of donated brains) has not been done. But, as I said earlier, CT scans and MRI scans show no evidence of obvious brain damage in people who stutter. It is just as likely that stuttering may involve something analogous to "crossed wires" in certain very specific brain areas (e.g. the SMA). Another important point is that there may be different causes in different people.

A Neuropsychological Theory of Stuttering
How Might Activity in the Right Hemisphere Affect Speech Fluency?

So far, I have talked about two different lines of evidence. The first one involves the relationship between the left and right cerebral hemispheres, and the tendency for greater activity in the right hemisphere of people who stutter than in fluent speakers. The second one involves the sequencing of complex movements. It is fairly easy to understand how the sequencing of complex movements might relate to speech fluency and stuttering. It is less obvious what a vaguely defined tendency for overactivity in the right hemisphere might have to do with stuttering. I must stress that we do not have a definitive answer to this question. We do, however, have some ideas, and I will share a few of those with you here.

I said earlier that the left and right hemispheres seem to be specialized for different functions. Speech and language, for example, are controlled mostly by the left cerebral hemisphere in most people. Emotions and spatial skills, on the other hand, are typically controlled more by the right hemisphere. I'd like to focus, for a moment, on emotions. It is well known to neuropsychologists and neurologists that *strong negative emotions like anxiety and fear are associated with activity in the right hemisphere in most people.* If people who stutter already have a tendency for greater right hemisphere activity than fluent speakers, then negative emotions might be expected to lead to even more right hemisphere activation in them than in fluent speakers. And it is clear that most people who stutter do experience those emotions in situations they associate with stuttering. Lise and Sally Bowman have described that aspect of stuttering very thoroughly.

For some people who stutter, just hearing the phone ring creates fear or dread. For others, it might be when they have to introduce themselves, or order food in a restaurant. Also, for many people, there are certain words and sounds that are particularly difficult for them. Consequently, these words and sounds may also become associated with fear and anxiety. Throughout my research, I have heard many stories from people who stutter about how they deal with these sounds and situations. As Lise and Sally Bowman have discussed, one approach is to avoid the difficult sound or situation. A lady I met recently told me a story about how she dealt with one very difficult school situation. At her Catholic girl's school, the students were required to stand and read their own test marks to the entire class. This lady recalled that she had particular problems with the "s" sound as a schoolgirl. Consequently, saying "sixty" or "seventy" was a great problem for her. She was obviously a very intelligent person, but when she couldn't guarantee getting marks in the eighties, she would "engineer" marks that would allow her to pass without facing the dreaded "s." That meant marks in the 50's.

There are very few people who stutter who would dispute that the experience of stuttering creates feelings of anxiety, frustration or even fear. It is also likely that, over time, many of those emotions may become "transferred" to the words, sounds or situations that trigger stuttering: the phone, the arrival of a waiter, or the classroom situation I described above, for example. The triggers themselves may be creating a situation that increases the tendency for right hemisphere activity in the person who stutters. But how does that activity affect speech? We believe there are at least two different ways that speech might be adversely affected by the greater right hemisphere activity in people who stutter.

First, that right hemisphere activity might "spill over" and interfere with the fragile speech-motor mechanisms that people who stutter seem to possess. The tendency for activity in one brain area to interfere with activity in another area is a well-known principle of human neuropsychology (this phenomenon can be illustrated by attempting to rub your stomach while patting your head). If activity originating in the right hemisphere spills over into the fragile speech-motor mechanisms, then those mechanisms would be more likely to experience momentary breakdowns. Those breakdowns would be experienced by the person as disruptions in the timing of his or her speech muscles: dysfluencies.

Second, activity in the right hemisphere may draw attentional resources away from the left hemisphere mechanisms that control speech and language under normal circumstances. Everyone has a limited pool of cognitive resources that they can draw upon to carry out the various "higher" brain functions. The excess right hemisphere activity associated with a person's "trigger" situations may be drawing resources away from the important and demanding task of controlling speech. This would place an additional burden on the speech mechanisms by leaving them with fewer resources to do their job.

I'd like to stress that there is no reason to assume that the greater right hemisphere activity apparent in people who stutter is a "weakness" of any kind. It is likely that there are many people who have a similar pattern of brain activity but who do not stutter. Who knows, it may just be that Isaac Newton (who stuttered) would never have uncovered the mysteries of planetary motion if his right hemisphere hadn't been as active as it was!

A Vicious Circle

Nevertheless, if the individual also has a speech-motor timing difficulty (as described above), then the stage appears to be set for a kind of vicious circle. It may start before the person even begins to speak. The phone rings, the waiter arrives, or the teacher beckons. That alone could increase the right hemisphere activity by creating feelings of fear or anxiety in the individual. Thus, the fragile speech-motor mechanisms in the brain are being subjected to a source of interference even before the first movement is initiated.

Recall that the brain area we suspect, the SMA, is very important for the initiation of complex movements. Interference from the right hemisphere to the SMA could essentially "sabotage" a new speech movement before it was uttered. As the speech attempt faltered, the individual would experience frustration as well as greater anxiety regarding the speaking situation. That would fuel even more right hemisphere activity, worsening the situation. A "struggle" would ensue – a vicious circle, or "snowball effect." In scientific terms, this is known as a "positive feedback loop." Positive feedback loops tend to get out of control! This vicious circle would explain how a very mild timing difficulty could be amplified to the point where speech is affected in a major way. The cycle is illustrated in the diagram below.

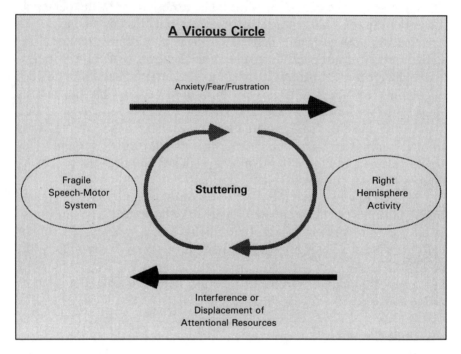

Anger: A Paradox?

Most people would consider anger to be a negative emotion. In general, anger *is* considered to be one of the emotions that are associated with right hemisphere activity. Why, then, do many people who stutter report that they stutter *less* when they are angry? For example, Lucas was very fluent while explaining why he was so angry at his grade seven science teacher.

Once again, we do not have any definitive answers to this question. There are, however, a couple of points worth mentioning. First, bouts of anger may in fact involve an increase in self-confidence (temporarily at least!). That increase in self-confidence may help the individual focus his resources on the task of speaking, rather than on whether or not he will be able to speak. Most people who stutter will be more fluent if they are distracted from the fact that they stutter. This is known to speech pathologists as the "distraction" effect. Remember that the "positive feedback loop" depends on the person being aware of their speech, and on the way dysfluencies will amplify frustration, fear or anxiety. Outwardly directed anger, even though it is a negative emotion, would not result in the same kind of cycle, because of the distraction effect. It is a negative emotion that is unrelated to the immediate act of speaking.

"Why Doesn't My Cousin Stutter When He Sings?"

Most people who stutter are either more fluent or perfectly fluent when they sing. There are a number of possible reasons for this. Singing involves some brain areas that are not involved in speech. Singing may also affect the overall pattern of activity between the two cerebral hemispheres differently than speaking. In addition, singing adds a "rhythm" to the person's voice, and this may assist in overcoming the subtle timing problem involved in stuttering. In Chapter One, Sally Bowman described a variety of accessory activities (finger snapping, foot stomping, etc.) associated with stuttering that may well represent conscious or subconscious attempts to do something similar.

Speech Therapy: How It Might Work

Speech therapy might work in two different ways. First, by teaching the person techniques to improve fluency (e.g. stretched syllables, full breath, gentle onsets), speech therapy helps to simplify the speech task. This makes it more resistant to the momentary breakdowns that can ultimately lead to more serious dysfluencies. With reference to the vicious circle, this is essentially like "nipping it in the bud." As these skills become more practiced, the "fragile" speech mechanisms in the brain become more resistant to interference from other brain activity.

Second, speech therapy may also help improve the person's confidence in the face of their "trigger" situations. As he develops confidence in his speech skills, he will be less likely to experience the negative emotions in those situations. That will mean less activation in the right hemisphere, and thus less interference with the fragile speech mechanisms. Some speech programs focus exclusively on the emotional aspect of stuttering. What success those programs have (usually short-lived) is probably rooted in their ability to "turn off the fuel" that interferes with the person's speech. Other speech therapy programs focus on the speech skills, but also address the emotional issues directly. But even programs that focus exclusively on speech skills will have an indirect affect on the emotional side by increasing the individual's confidence in his or her ability to speak fluently in any situation.

Auditory Feedback and Masking Devices

One area of research I have conspicuously neglected is the work on auditory (hearing) processes in stuttering. In short, a variety of devices (that have been mentioned by Lise) have been shown to improve fluency by either blocking or delaying auditory feedback to the person who is speaking. There are many different theories as to how these devices work. One possibility is that the altered feedback serves to break the "positive feedback loop" I described with respect to the speech mechanisms and right hemisphere activation. If the individual cannot hear himself speaking, then the source of information that may be fuelling his anxiety (and hence right hemisphere activation) is blocked.

Recovery in Children

Not all children who stutter will continue to stutter into adulthood. In fact, approximately 75% of children who stutter will stop stuttering before reaching adolescence. Most will stop stuttering within a year or two from when they start stuttering. Unfortunately, it is currently very difficult for speech therapists to predict which children are, and which children are not, going to continue to stutter as adolescents and adults. Perhaps if we understood why some children seem to just "grow out of" their stutter, we could develop a means to predict who will recover and who won't. We might even be in a better position to help those who wouldn't otherwise be expected to recover.

It may be that some forms of stuttering are related to the immaturity of the young speaker's brain. Some parts of the brain do not mature fully until late childhood or early adolescence. In particular, it is well known that two areas of the brain, known as the corpus callosum and the frontal lobes, are among the last to reach maturity. The SMA is a part of our frontal lobe, and also has important connections that go through the corpus callosum. This means that there are almost certainly aspects of the SMA's functions that don't reach maturity until late childhood or early adolescence. People whose SMA is perfectly normal, but who have a tendency for overactivity in the right hemisphere, might be expected to stutter as children, because their speech mechanisms are immature. However, they would be expected to stop stuttering as the relevant brain structures reached a sufficient level of maturation.

A Closing Note

I hope it is clear by now why both psychology and neurology are important to understanding stuttering. Whether or not the theory I have described is correct, two things are clear. First, stuttering has a neurological cause. Second, the expression of stuttering is influenced by emotional factors. Since we also know that emotions are related to the functioning of our brain, we must at least attempt to explore the relationship between those emotions and the neurological cause of stuttering.

One final comment. The theory I have described here attributes stuttering to neurological mechanisms that we are not in a position to "cure" today. However, psychological factors are extremely important to the expression of stuttering. People who stutter develop the fears and frustrations they associate with stuttering only with the willing contribution of our society – a society that treats stuttering as a sign of weakness, a reason for guilt, and a source of humour. A change in the attitude of that society might be the best "pill" one could prescribe for people who stutter. Hopefully this book will help to promote that change.

*　　*　　*

David Forster is a doctoral student studying neuropsychology at Carleton University in Ottawa, Canada. He has a Master of Science degree in psychology, and has been studying the neuropsychology of stuttering with Dr. William Webster since 1988. His specific interest in his doctoral work has been the role of brain development in the spontaneous recovery that many children who stutter experience. He also has a personal interest in stuttering; his younger brother Robin stutters.

REFERENCE GUIDE TO TREATMENT CENTRES AND OTHER RESOURCES

There are highly effective treatment programs available for people who stutter. Listed below are some of the successful centres operating in Canada and in the United States.

CANADIAN CLINICS

Department of Speech Pathology and Audiology, Jill Harrison, M.Sc., S-LP (C) (Adult programme but teens from age 17 and up are also accepted) The Montréal General Hospital, 1650 Cedar Avenue, Montréal, Québec H3G 1A4, **(514) 934-8028, (514) 937-6011.**

André Courcy, M.O.A.
Orthophonistes, Prévention – Evaluation – Intervention, Enfants – Adolescents – Adultes, (Services offerts en français), 200 ouest, boulevard Saint-Joseph, Montréal (Québec) H2T 2P8, **(514) 273-3613.**

Rosalee Shenker, Ph.D., S-LP
The Fluency Centre, 5735 Monkland Avenue, Montréal, Québec H4A 1E7, **(514) 489-2238.** Rosalee Shenker and her associate, Glenna Waters, offer bilingual and intensive treatment sessions as well as special teen programs.

Chantale Tremblay, M.O.A.
Orthophoniste, (services offerts en français), 360 ouest, boulevard Saint-Joseph, Montréal (Québec) H2V 2N9, **(514) 272-5900),** (514) 271-6752 (télécopieur).

Communication Disorders
(Treatment program for adults and adolescents.) The Rehabilitation Centre, Royal Ottawa Health Care Group, 505 Smyth Road, Ottawa, Ontario K1H 8M2, **(613) 739-5302,** (613) 737-7056 (fax).

Karen Luker, M.H.Sc., SLP(C)
Speech-Language Pathologist, 1 Saddle Crescent, Ottawa, Ontario K1G 5L4, **(613) 739-4376.**

Susan Glazer, M.Sc., Reg. OSLA, SLP(C)
Centrepointe Professional Services, 98 Centrepointe Drive, Nepean, Ontario K2G 6B1, **(613) 228-1174,** (613) 228-2756 (fax). Susan provides a full range of speech therapy services for children and adolescents with articulation, language, stuttering and voice disorders.

Medd Shane Theoret-Douglas & Associates Inc.

Speech-Language Pathologists, Reg. OSLA, SLP(C), Reg. CASLPO. In addition to individual therapy, MSTD offers monthly maintenance group sessions for youngsters aged 6-16 who have learned and are attempting to generalize and maintain fluency facilitating techniques. Receipts are issued for refund through private insurance coverage. P.O. Box 473, Orléans, Ontario K1C 1S8, **(613) 830-5963** (East Ottawa), **(613) 835-4174** (South/East Ottawa), **(613) 228-7140** (West/Central).

Robert M. Kroll, Ph.D., Reg. OSLA

Head of the Speech Pathology Department, Clarke Institute of Psychiatry, 250 College Street, Toronto, Ontario M5T 1R8, **(416) 979-2221.**

KIDSPEECH (4 locations)

720 Sheppard Avenue, Suite 6, Pickering, Ontario, L1V 1G5
19 Larabee Crescent, Don Mills, Ontario M3A 3E6
596 Kingston Road West, Ajax, Ontario L1T 3A2
4581 Highway #7, Suite 105, Unionville, Ontario L3R 1M6
(416) 44-SPEAK OR (416) 447-7325, (416) 391-4078 (fax).

Institute for Stuttering Treatment and Research (ISTAR)

Affiliated with the University of Alberta. Executive Director: Einer Boberg, Ph.D., S-SP(C), CCC-Sp., #401, 8540-109 Street, Edmonton, Alberta T6G 1E6, **(403) 492-2619,** (403) 492-8457 (fax).

Calgary Health Services

Varina Russell, M.Sc., (A), S-LP(C), Reg., (Alta), Director, Speech-Language Pathology Division, Northwest Health Centre, #109, 1829 Ranchlands Blvd., N.W., Calgary, Alberta T3G 2A7, **(403) 241-0063,** (403) 239-6056 (fax).

U.S. CLINICS

Geneseo

Starbuck Fluency Enhancing Clinics

Kathleen R. Jones, Ph.D., CCC-Sp, Administrative Program Director (Family, Child, Adolescent, and Adult Programs: Residential and Intensive) Department of Speech Pathology, State University of New York at Geneseo. One College Circle, Geneseo, New York 14454, **(716) 245-5332.**

Catherine S. Otto, M.S., CCC-SLP

Director, Total Immersion Fluency Training, 27 West 20th Street, Suite 1203, New York, New York 10011, **(212) 633-6400.**

Richard Forcucci, Ph.D.

Leader Clinic, Edinboro University of Pennsylvania, Edinboro, Pennsylvannia 16444, **(814) 732-2433.**

Dorvan H. Breitenfeldt, Ph.D.

Coordinator, Stuttering Workshop, SSMP (Successful Stuttering Management Program). Three-week summer workshop and a manual of the program is available for purchase. Eastern Washington University, School of Health Services, Department of Communication Disorders, MS-106, 108 Communications Building, Cheney, Washington 99004-2495, **(509) 359-6622**, (509) 359-6802 (fax) or (509) 359-6927 (fax).

Hollins Communications Research Institute

Ronald L. Webster, Ph.D., Director, Hollins Fluency System (TM), 19-day intensive treatment program, (originator: The Precision Fluency Shaping Program), P.O. Box 9737, Roanoke, VA 24020, **(703) 362-6528.**

The Precision Fluency Shaping Program (PFSP)

Ross S. Barrett, M.A. CCC-SLP. Eastern Virginia Medical School, 855 West Brambleton Avenue, Norfolk, Virginia 23510, **(804) 446-5938.**

Carl W. Dell Jr. Ph.D.

Speech and Hearing Clinic, Eastern Illinois University, Charleston, IL 61920, **(217) 581-2712.**

Stanley Goldberg, Ph.D.

Director, Center for Interdisciplinary Clinical Studies, Department of Special Education, San Francisco State University, 1600 Holloway Avenue, San Francisco, CA 94132, **(415) 338-6196**, (415) 338-0566 (fax).

Sally Bowman, M.S., CCC-SLP

Camp Director and Associate Professor Emeritus, Indiana University, School of Medicine, Department of Otolaryngology, Riley Hospital 0860, 702 Barnhill Drive, Indianapolis, Indiana 46202-5230, **(317) 630-8966; (317) 274-8868** or **(317) 630-8915** (317) 630-8958 (fax).

SUMMER PROGRAMS

Fluency Training Through Family Involvement

Dick Mallard, Ph.D., Communicative Disorders Program, Southwest Texas State University, 601 University Drive, San Marcos, TX 78666-4616, **(512) 245-2344.** (Students do NOT direct this program; all therapy is coordinated by experienced professionals.)

Shady Trails Camp
  University of Michigan, 1111 East Catherine Street, Ann Arbor, MI
  48109-2054, **(313) 764-8442** Voice/TDD, (313) 747-2489 (fax).

Summer Remedial Clinics
  (for children 6-17 years), Central Michigan University, Laura A.
  McBride, M.A., CCC-SLP, Director, Moore Hall, 441, CMU, Mt. Pleasant, MI 48859, **(517) 774-3472** and **(571) 774-7294.**

OTHER SOURCES OF INFORMATION

Canadian Association for People Who Stutter (CAPS)
  Attention: Jaan Pill, 228 Galloway Road, Suite 309, Scarborough, Ontario, Canada M1E 5G6, **(416) 286-4363,** (416) 286-5779 (fax).

International Fluency Association (IFA), Attention: Einer Boberg, Ph.D.
  Institute for Stuttering Treatment and Research, #401, 8540-109 Street,
  Edmonton, Alberta, Canada T6G 1E6, **(403) 492-2619,** (403) 492-8457
  (fax).

Speak Easy, Inc.
  (Canada's national charitable organization for people who stutter, parents of children who stutter, professionals in the field, and the general
  public. Speak Easy publishes an informative monthly magazine and as-
  sists in the formation of local community support groups.) Mike Hugues,
  Executive Director, 95 Evergreen Avenue, St. John, New Brunswick,
  Canada E2N 1H4, **(506) 696-6799.**

Association des bègues du Canada Inc. (ABC)
  (Bulletin *COMMUNIQUER* – réunions hebdomadaires), 7801, rue Ste-
  Claire, Montréal (Québec), Canada H1L 1V8, **(514) 353-1042** et **(514)
  649-0863.**

Speechmasters of Ottawa
  Self-Help Group for People Who Stutter: weekly meetings, quarterly
  newsletter: *THE VOICE MONITOR,* c/o The Communication Disorders
  Department, The Rehabilitation Centre, 505 Smyth Road, Ottawa, Ontario, Canada K1H 8M2, **(613) 739-5302,** (613) 737-7056 (fax) or you
  may contact: Richard Inomata, President, 2063 Wildflower Drive,
  Orléans, Ontario, Canada K1E 3R4, **(613) 995-7841 (W), (613) 830-1710
  (h);** or Norm McEwen, Past President, 29 Brent Avenue, Nepean, Ontario, Canada K2G 3L1, **(613) 957-1732 (w), (613) 226-7001(h).**

Stuttering Association of Toronto (SAT)

Attention: Jacob Aharon, 312 Dolomite Drive, Suite 205, Downsview, Ontario, Canada M3J 2N2, **(416) 650-5110,** (416) 650-6142 (fax).

The British Columbia Association of People Who Stutter

Vancouver Chapter, *B.C. Blockbuster* published 3 times per annum. Don Hermansen, 150 April Road, Port Moody, British Columbia Canada V3H 3M6, **(604) 469-1282,** (604) 469-1257 (fax).

The Stuttering Foundation of America

(They offer a whole range of wonderful books and brochures on stuttering; also videotapes and referral network), P.O. Box 11749, Memphis, TN 38111-0749, **(800) 992-9392.**

Aaron's Associates

Excellent newsletter for young children who stutter; published throughout school year. Editor: Janice Westbrook, Ph.D., M.Ed., CCC-SP, 6114 Waterway, Garland, Texas 75043 U.S.A., **(214) 226-9855.**

National Stuttering Project (NSP)

John Ahlbach, Executive Director. Informative monthly newsletter *Letting Go* and many other publications available through this non-profit organization, 208-2151 Irving Street, San Francisco, CA 94122-1609, **(415) 566-5324,** (415) 664-3721 (fax), **(800) 364-1677.**

INFORMATION ON THE VIDEO *Speaking of Courage:*

Purchases can be made through Magic Lantern Communication Ltd., #38-775 Pacific Road, Oakville, Ontario L6L 6M4; Canada East toll free number: 1-800-263-1717; Canada West toll free number: 1-800-263-1818.

BIBLIOGRAPHY

Bondarenko, V. 1993. *Speaking of Courage* Documentary. Magic Lantern Communications Ltd., Distributor, Video: 60 minutes.

Bowman, S. 1983. *What Everyone Should Know About Stuttering.* Bowman & Associates, Booklet: 20 Pages.

Carlisle, J.A. 1985. *Tangled Tongue.* University of Toronto Press. 258 pages.

Cloutier-Steele, L.G. 1992. *The Ontario Barber Shop Singers Harmonize for Speech,* Abilities. Canada's *Lifestyle Magazine for People With Disabilities.* Issue Number 11, Article. p. 116.

Dell. C. Jr. 1979. Reprinted in 1983, 1986, 1989 and 1991. *Treating the School Age Stutterer: A Guide for Clinicians.* Stuttering Foundation of America. Publication Number 14, 110 pages.

Fullerton, D.H. 1980. *Submission on Stuttering,* presented to the Special Parliamentary Committee on the Disabled and the Handicapped. Paper. 5 pages.

Mazzuca-Peter, J. *The Student Who Stutters: Some Questions and Answers.* Metropolitan Separate School Board Publication. Curriculum Resource Department. Article, 5 pages.

Webster, W.G. and Marie G. Poulos. 1989. *Facilitating Fluency: Transfer Strategies for Adult Stuttering Treatment Programs.* Communication Skill Builders, Inc. 86 pages.

Westbrook, J. 1993. *Fluency Aids.* The Staff Newsletter. Aaron's Associates. Article, 2 pages.

INDEX

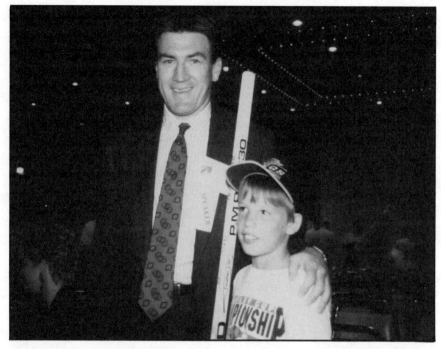

Lucas with Dave Taylor of the L.A. Kings hockey team at the meeting of the National Stuttering Project in San Francisco.